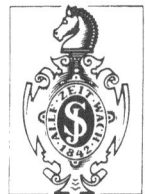

Holger Pettersson · Marvin Gilbert

Diagnostic Imaging in Hemophilia

Musculoskeletal and Other Hemorrhagic
Complications

With 102 Figures

Springer-Verlag
Berlin Heidelberg New York Tokyo

Holger Pettersson, MD
Associate Professor of Radiology, University of Lund, Sweden
Head, Division for Skeletal Radiology, Department of Radiology,
University Hospital, Lund, Sweden

Marvin S. Gilbert, MD
Associate Clinical Professor, Department of Orthopedics, Mt. Sinai
School of Medicine, City University of New York, U.S.A.

ISBN-13:978-1-4471-1374-4   e-ISBN-13:978-1-4471-1372-0
DOI: 10.1007/978-1-4471-1372-0

Library of Congress Cataloging in Publication Data
Pettersson, Holger, 1942–
Diagnostic imaging in hemophilia.
Includes bibliographies and index. 1. Hemophilia—Complications and sequelae—
Diagnostic. 2. Hemorrhage—Diagnosis. 3. Musculoskeletal system—Radiography.
4. Diagnosis, Radioscopic. 5. Imaging systems in medicine. I. Gilbert, Marvin, 1939–
II. Title.
DNLM: 1. Hemophilia—complications. 2. Hemophilia—radiography. WH 325 P499d
RC642.P48 1985 616.1′572 85-2568
ISBN-13:978-1-4471-1374-4(U.S.)

© by Springer-Verlag Berlin Heidelberg 1985
Softcover reprint of the hardcover 1st edition 1985

Filmset and printed by
BAS Printers Limited, Over Wallop, Stockbridge, Hampshire

2128/3916-543210

to Grethe, Christina and Anders
and Maxine, Cynthia and Richard

Preface

During recent decades there has been a revolutionary change in the life expectancy and quality of life of the hemophiliac. This has been achieved by hematologic and clinical research, and the future for the hemophiliac depends upon further medical knowledge and research.

In spite of the dramatically improved life situation of hemophiliacs, hemorrhagic complications remain a threat. The hemorrhagic disorder may influence and/or aggravate the course of trauma or other diseases in these patients. Hemophiliacs suffering from hemorrhagic complications or eligible for elective surgery should be referred to Hemophilia Treatment and Training Centers, where evaluation and examination are performed by a multidisciplinary team with experience and interest in the disease. The radiologist is an important member of this team.

In the past diagnostic imaging has been based mainly on conventional radiography, and this is still very important for the diagnosis of hemophilic complications, but the diagnostic imaging of today offers a wide range of modalities—conventional radiography, computed tomography, sonography, radionuclide imaging, and, in its infancy, magnetic resonance imaging. Thus there is a need for a thorough description of the potential and limitations of these modern diagnostic techniques.

Owing to modern technical development, present-day diagnostic imaging has a wide potential and provides important contributions in two principally different situations:

1. In the diagnostic workup of hemorrhagic complications, diagnostic imaging may provide the foundation for correct clinical assessment and proper decisions regarding treatment. It has an important role in the differential diagnosis of CNS or intra-abdominal bleeding and in the planning of orthopedic surgery. In these situations, diagnostic imaging has proven to be an invaluable tool in the diagnostic arsenal.

2. Modern treatment is expensive and has many inherited risks, as discussed in the following chapter. Therefore, it is very important to evaluate the cost-effectiveness of modern treatment, in terms of both economy and complications of treatment. In this respect, diagnostic imaging may provide objective information on the effect of treatment of hemophilic

arthropathy, and radiologic examination is an important parameter in several ongoing national and international investigations on this topic.

Therefore, any physician, pediatrician, internist, hematologist, or orthopedic surgeon involved in the treatment of a hemophiliac, be it in the physician's office or as part of a multidisciplinary treatment team, should be able to assess the information provided by diagnostic imaging examinations. Similarly, the radiologist involved must be versed in the problems and participate in the discussions of the clinicians. This mutual understanding and cooperation is the solid foundation for proper management of the hemophilic patient, and it is the authors' hope that the present book will provide a basis for such understanding.

This book is the result of such multidisciplinary cooperation. The first chapter has been written by the Directors and a member of two leading International Hemophilia Treatment and Training Centers—those of Mount Sinai Hospital, The City University of New York, U.S.A. and The General Hospital of Malmö, University of Lund, Sweden. It is intended to introduce the reader who is less familiar with hemophilic problems into the concepts of the disease, its demography, its complications, and the problems of modern, effective treatment.

Because the majority of bleeding episodes occur within the musculoskeletal system, the orthopedic surgeon serves as Codirector of the Center at Mount Sinai Hospital, and the following chapters are jointly written by this orthopedic surgeon (M.G.) and by the radiologist who has been responsible for and had long experience with hemophilic problems at The General Hospital of Malmö (H.P.). The comments on radionuclide imaging have been provided by the Head of the Nuclear Medicine Division at another leading center, The Hospital for Sick Children, Toronto, Canada.

After a presentation of modern diagnostic imaging, the reader is given a detailed description of the hemorrhagic complications as they appear in diagnostic imaging, as well as the clinical course and the pathologic findings. Musculoskeletal problems are emphasized, but hemorrhage into the central nervous system and the body cavities, although less common, may be a serious threat to the patient, and is given due consideration.

It is the authors' hope that this book will provide the reader with a single source of insight and knowledge, allowing all medical professionals involved in the care of hemophiliacs to proceed towards our common goal: a better life for our patients.

Lomma, Sweden   Holger Pettersson
1985   Marvin Gilbert

Acknowledgements

We wish to express our sincere gratitude and appreciation to the following institutions and people:

Olle Olssons Research Fund and Travenol Laboratories for valuable financial support.

The secretaries, in particular Mona Helleberg and Mona Olsson, for enthusiastic and conscientious work.

The photographer, Göran Eliasson, for skilful and very professional help.

Our colleagues and partners for allowing us to take time away from our work to prepare this manuscript.

In addition, the first section of Chapter 1, by Louis M. Aledort, was supported in part by HSA grant ♯MCB-360001-04-01, Regional Comprehensive Hemophilia Diagnostic and Treatment Center, The Margie Boas Fund, and the Polly Annenberg Levee Hematology Center, Department of Medicine at the Mt. Sinai School of Medicine of the City University of New York.

Contents

Contributors

Louis M. Aledort, MD
Professor and Vice Chairman,
Department of Medicine,
Mt. Sinai School of Medicine,
City University of New York, U.S.A.

David Gilday, MD, FRCP(C)
Associate Professor of Radiology,
University of Toronto, Canada
Head, Division of Nuclear Medicine,
Department of Radiology,
The Hospital for Sick Children,
Toronto, Ontario, Canada

S. Anders Larsson, MD
Assistant Professor of Surgery,
Surgical Registrar,
Department of Surgery,
General Hospital of Malmö,
University of Lund, Sweden

Inga Marie Nilsson, MD
Professor and Chairman,
Department of Coagulation Disorders,
General Hospital of Malmö,
University of Lund, Sweden

Chapter 1
The Disease

Hematologic Considerations—Past and Present
Louis M. Aledort

Although hemophilia was described early by the Egyptians and in the Talmud, it still remains a topic of great interest and excitement and a continued source of clinical investigation. The hemophilias are now recognized to be genetically transmitted disorders characterized by the inability to produce normal functioning coagulation factors. The lack of coagulation factors leads to spontaneous bleeding, particularly in those patients with severe disease. The bleeding, which is mainly into joint spaces, leads to marked alterations in joint function that in turn result in significant morbidity. Mortality from this disease has progressively decreased but remains a major challenge.

Definition

The hemophilias refer to three coagulation defects: factor VIII, factor IX, and factor XI deficiency. Factors VIII and IX are inherited as X-linked recessive patterns; factor XI is autosomal dominant with varying degrees of penetration. Deficiency of factors VIII (hemophilia A) and IX (hemophilia B) is clinically identical and the severity of the disease is correlated to the level of deficiency. Factor XI deficiency is much more capricious, the level of deficiency not always correlating with the severity of bleeding. The normal population has between 50% and 150% of any factor, and deficiencies are categorized as mild ($>5\%$), moderate (1%–5%), or severe ($<1\%$). The critical level of factor necessary for hemostasis, whether surgical or traumatic, is 30%. Patients with deficiencies between 30% and 50% are asymptomatic, can frequently withstand surgical intervention, but are genetically hemophiliacs and will pass on the genes despite their lack of clinical involvement. Factor XI deficiency is usually clinically mild even when severe at laboratory testing and rarely poses problems for the clinician. Its identification, however, is important because the patient may bleed at the time of surgical intervention. The factor VIII and IX deficiencies differ, in that patients with levels of less than 1% almost always experience significant hemorrhage.

Clinical Symptoms

Hemorrhage usually occurs spontaneously, and is particularly frequent into diarthrodial joints. The average number of bleeding episodes is approximately 35 a year in a severe hemophiliac. Repeated hemarthroses cause progressive destruction of the joints, and this hemophilic arthropathy, although not life threatening, does lead to severe disability. If one looks at the spectrum of the disease, the mild and moderate hemophiliacs bleed less often, some almost never, and their bleeding episodes are quite variable.

Although hemorrhage occurs most frequently into the joint spaces it also occurs into the soft tissues of the extremities, the trunk, and the body cavities. Soft tissue bleeding producing neuropathy is not infrequent. Retroperitoneal hematomas may be extensive and cause severe blood loss. On occasion they can lead to obstructive uropathy. Bleeding into the genitourinary tract is not uncommon but it rarely causes extensive blood loss and is seldom life threatening. Gastrointestinal hemorrhage is fortunately uncommon, but when it does occur it is a major problem in that there is no potential for tamponade. The most life-threatening site of bleeding is the central nervous system. Such hemorrhage remains the major cause of death in these patients. Thus in a recent survey 68% of all deaths in American hemophiliacs occurred from spontaneous hemorrhage, the most common form being into the central nervous system.

Development of Modern Treatment

As noted above, hemophilia as a clinical entity and its genetics were defined in the third century Talmud. However, the significance of hemophilia and its impact on society was underscored by the family of Queen Victoria. The transmission of the disease to the royal houses of Spain and Russia led many to regard it mistakenly as a "royal disease." At that time there was no control for the pain and bleeding associated with hemophilia, and it has been hypothesized that Rasputin gained influence with the Russian royal family because he was able to control the symptoms of the Czarevich by hypnosis. However, hemophilia from the time of Victoria until the mid 1900s remained a medical curiosity. The book *Nicholas and Alexandra*, written by the parents of a hemophiliac, dramatized and made public the problems that a hemophilic child causes for the family unit.

In the natural course of the disease, the pain of the initial hemarthrosis is followed by the pain of severe arthritis. In the past little if anything could be done other than immobilization of the joints. Dr. Henry Jordan, an orthopedic surgeon in New York, was a major force in this method of treatment. He used casting to correct flexion contractures and then immobilized both upper and lower extremities in braces to prevent further bleeding and deformity. Surgical intervention was impossible. Many patients died of either spontaneous hemorrhage or of diseases that were not associated with the hemorrhagic disorder but would have responded to surgical intervention.

In the 1940s major laboratory advances were made and it became clear that hemophiliacs were missing a plasmatic factor. Within a short period of time it became possible to differentiate factor VIII, IX, and XI deficiency in the laboratory. With a definite diagnosis it now became possible to consider definitive treatment. The introduction of blood banking ushered in the era of modern therapy for hemophilia. With the ability to separate red blood cells from plasma and the recognition that hemophilia factors were contained in the plasma, treatment became a reality. Fresh-frozen plasma could be administered intravenously to prevent life-threatening and crippling hemorrhages. The limitation of this treatment was experienced when intensive therapy was required. Plasma overload could lead to congestive heart failure and possibly death. This was particularly critical when surgical hemostasis was attempted. The mere loss of primary teeth and dental extractions necessitated long-term hospitalizations that were costly to society and to the patient.

The next major advance was made in the late 1960s when Judith Pool introduced cryoprecipitate. Working in Palo Alto, she serendipitously discovered that when plasma was rapidly frozen and then slowly thawed at 4°C a cryoprecipitate would form at the bottom of the plasma. This small portion of the plasma contained approximately 50% of the factor VIII present in the original plasma. The problem of vascular overload had been solved. Almost immediately following this, the plasma fractionators, a major force in the treatment of hemophilia, were able to fractionate the cryoprecipitate further and to prepare it in a lyophilized form. The residual plasma could also be further fractionated for factor IX. These two products, known as "concentrates," have become the mainstay of hemophilia therapy throughout the world.

Between the late 1960s and the mid 1970s many companies entered the field of plasma fractionation and the technology improved significantly. From 1975 on there was a more than adequate supply of factor VIII and factor IX to meet the needs of hemophiliacs. These fractions, powdered, easy to dissolve, and reconstituted in small volumes, could be easily administered intravenously so that hemostatic levels could be reached and maintained without difficulty for long periods of time. A major effort could therefore be made to analyze and try to prevent the chronic problems that faced the hemophiliac. Orthopedic and oral surgical intervention could be undertaken without undue risk. As these problems were being solved, many of the nonmedical aspects of hemophilia took on greater importance. It was during this era that comprehensive care was developed as a method of treatment.

The first comprehensive program was developed at the Los Angeles Orthopedic Hospital under the guidance of Dr. Shelby Dietrich. Within a short time a multidisciplinary clinical comprehensive care program was started at the Mount Sinai Hospital. These programs have become models for hemophilic care throughout the world. In addition they serve as models for comprehensive care of other chronic diseases. Innovations in health care delivery, medical management, and psychosocial issues can be and are constantly evaluated within these models. The multidisciplinary team should include the following personnel: a primary physician such as an internist or a pediatrician, a hematologist, an orthopedic surgeon, a physical therapist, a dentist, an oral surgeon, a vocational rehabilitation counsellor, a psychiatrist, a social worker, a neurologist, a radiologist, and a nurse clinician. Educational programs for patients, family, and community are essential. In 1976 the U.S. government provided funds to develop a network of intermeshing comprehensive care programs so that all patients within the country could be cared for.

Concomitant with these advances there was a critical change in the way in which a factor was delivered to the patient. This modality was that of self-infusion or "home care." Dr. Benjamin Alexander in Boston was the first physician to infuse a patient with a plasma at the patient's home. This manner of treatment was discontinued because of a high incidence of transfusion reactions. A second trial was started in Rochester and discontinued for the same reason. However, in the early 1970s there was renewed interest in the possibility of self-care, particularly as concentrates were now available. This time the program proved successful and within a short time this concept swept the country and guidelines for self-infusion were written by the National Hemophilia Foundation. Self-therapy has become a critical part of comprehensive care throughout the world. At first there was much resistance to this because of the problem of allowing the patient to participate in his own treatment by making therapeutic decisions, but with more experience it became clear that with careful patient and family selection, a superb modality of therapy had evolved.

In most programs, whether they involve self-treatment or treatment at a Hemophilia Center, factor replacement is given on demand, i.e., there is early treatment for bleeding episodes. In some centers another regimen is used, especially in children and young adults. These patients are given prophylaxis, which is replacement therapy given regularly every 2nd–4th day to prevent or reduce the number of bleeding episodes. The effect of this modality is presently being evaluated.

Another key advance in the management of hemophilia has come from the study of bleeding problems in the oral cavity. In this area increased fibrinolytic activity is present and this leads to prolonged bleeding in patients with coagulation disorders. With the advent of replacement therapy it became possible to carry out oral surgical procedures but about 14 days of factor replacement was necessary. This entailed long-term hospitalization and high cost for simple therapeutic procedures. In the early 1970s work was done by an English group and then corroborated in America. These researches showed that by the addition of an inhibitor of fibrinolysis, such as transamenic acid or ε-aminocaproic acid, one could almost eliminate the need for long-term replacement therapy. With this adjunctive therapy many surgical procedures could be done outside the hospital with only minor complications.

Complications of Therapy

In 1975 a conference was held under the aegis of the National Heart Lung and Blood Institute, the Bureau of Biologics, and the National Hemophilia Foundation. At that conference the complications of transfusion therapy were outlined in detail.

Inhibitors

Approximately 15% of all hemophilia patients with factor VIII deficiency develop inhibitors. They occur early, and are especially frequent in patients with severe disease. In factor IX deficiency the frequency of inhibitor formation is much less. The inhibitor represents a significant clinical challenge for it frequently eliminates the effectiveness of the replacement therapy. During the prospective National Heart Lung and Blood Institute study which lasted from 1975 to 1979 it became apparent that there were two types of inhibitor patients:

1. Those who had little anamnestic response to repeated doses of factor VIII and who could achieve normal hemostasis with increased levels of factor replace-

ment. Approximately 25% of the patients fell into this group. These patients are called "low responders."

2. The remainder were "high responders" in that the inhibitor level increased dramatically following factor VIII infusion. This made replacement therapy essentially impossible, and these patients consequently became major therapeutic problems. In the mid 1970s it became clear that ordinary factor IX concentrates had the ability, in some cases, to bypass this inhibitor activity. A random double-blind prospective study was carried out which showed that 50% of bleeding episodes could be successfully treated in this manner. Following this, due to innovations from the fractionation industry, activated factor IX products became available which were capable of effectively stopping major bleeding episodes in many resistant patients. However, these products are quite expensive, and they have increased the cost of managing patients with inhibitors as compared with the cost when inhibitors are not used. Improved porcine factor VIII concentrates can also be successfully used to treat patients with low titer antibodies who have anamnestic responses. No substantial cross-reactivity with porcine factor VIII has been found in these patients. Attempts to induce immune intolerance by continuous high dose factor VIII infusion for long periods, accompanied in some cases by factor IX products, have been reported as successful at several centers. The costs associated with eliminating the inhibitor in this manner are, however, staggering.

These modalities of therapy, which are quite exciting, represent the beginning of an era of research that may prove very rewarding. The future direction for inhibitor management is to develop cheaper, better, more specific bypassing activity substances, as well as to define those patients who will develop inhibitors, define the inhibitor state such that it might be prevented, and possibly to eradicate the inhibitor once it is formed.

Immune Hemolysis

Most factor VIII concentrates, and cryoprecipitate plasma, contain anti-A and anti-B antibodies. Patients receiving large quantities of these materials, particularly in the surgical setting, have a propensity for immune hemolysis. Perusal of the peripheral blood during their administration usually reveals spherocytosis concomitant with hemolysis. It is not common for the hemolytic process to become significant enough to produce a severe anemia, but when it does, this can be overcome by the transfusion of type O blood. Some fractionators have produced type-specific factors and these are effective. Recipients of factor IX concentrates do not develop hemolysis.

Viral Transmission

Prior to hepatitis B testing all fractions contained hepatitis B virus. With the advent of hepatitis B testing it appears that hepatitis B transmission has been reduced but that not all carriers have been eliminated. Hepatitis B is still transmitted, but at a much lower incidence, i.e., approximately 8% a year. On the other hand non-A non-B hepatitis remains a major problem in factor concentrates today. Currently in our patient population approximately 50% show elevation of SGOT or SGPT, 5%–7% show persistence of the B antigenemia, and 90% have B markers. High dose cryoprecipitate recipients have similar markers. There is controversy as to whether recipients of low doses of cryoprecipitate have fewer markers. This question has not yet been totally resolved.

As early as 1975 it became clear that patients who developed elevation of their liver enzymes, whether persistent or not, could develop liver disease. Multiple studies have been carried out and the largest study, a prospective international cooperative study of 155 liver biopsies, revealed that the incidence of cirrhosis and/or chronic active hepatitis in the population studied was approximately 25%. In 1975 the mortality from liver disease was less than 1%, but currently it appears that it has increased to approximately 9% and may become one of the major causes of death in hemophilia. Epstein-Barr, cytomegalo- and parvo-viruses also appear to be commonly transmitted in factor concentrates. Their relationship to liver disease is just beginning to be studied.

Immune Complexes

It is apparent that a large percentage of patients with hemophilia have immune aberrations with elevated immune complexes as well as elevated immune globulins. The importance of these immune complexes and elevated globulins and their relationship to liver disease and AIDS remains unclear.

AIDS

In March 1982 the first case of hemophilia with acquired immune deficiency syndrome (AIDS) was diagnosed. What hemophiliacs had in common with other patients who had developed AIDS (heroin addicts and homosexuals) was that they all had elevated immune complexes, and a similar incidence of Australian antigen positivity as well as B markers. In addition, they were lymphopenic and had reversed T helper/T suppressor cell ratios. Within a short time, multiclinic studies revealed that anywhere from 50% to 70% of patients with hemophilia have T cell aberrations. These markers appear in those on high dose therapy, whether cryoprecipitate or fractions are used. No differences are seen with plasma derived from volunteer or paid blood. The reversal of the T cell ratio is due to an increase in suppressor cells. These patients are asymptomatic, although the syndrome of idopathic thrombocytopenic purpura and herpes zoster has been described.

In the hemophiliacs with AIDS, the reversal of T cell ratio is substantially different. In these there is a marked decrease in both Ts and Th with a reversal. In contrast to the homosexuals and the heroin addicts, the hemophiliacs with AIDS have only had opportunistic infections, the most prominent being *Pneumocystis carinii*. The findings in these hemophiliacs coupled with the similarities to the other high risk groups have supported a currently held theory that AIDS is a blood-borne viral illness. An alternate theory is that the chronic exposure to infectious agents plus chronic antigen overload are the causes of immune deficiency, which then leads to opportunistic infection and/or Kaposi sarcoma in AIDS patients.

Recent Advances

After years of work, fractionators have now produced altered factor material which has a reduced viral content. Clinical investigations show that they may alter the transmission of B and non-A non-B hepatitis. Within the next year all manufacturers will have viral "reduced" products. These factors are clearly effective, retaining normal biologic activity. However, until clinical trials are carried out, we will not know how effectively they reduce the transmission of viral diseases. There is also concern that an altered antigen state may occur which may produce more inhibitors. We are also worried about their cost-effectiveness. These products cost more, and more source plasma is needed. We must know whether they lead to less viral infections. On the other hand, the products are a major step forward in attempting to eliminate or reduce some of the complications of transfusion therapy. A prospective multicenter study is needed to solve some of these issues.

Recently a major and most exciting new event has taken place in the armamentarium of hemophilia therapy. 1-desamino-8-D-arginine vasodesmopressin acetate (DDAVP) is a vasopressin analogue that has the capability of raising the factor level in patients with mild and moderate hemophilia A and von Willebrand's disease. It can thus diminish the need for transfusion therapy. In addition, in Sweden it has been used in normal blood donors to raise plasma factor VIII level to increase the retrieval from source plasma. It is our hope that DDAVP will become an international therapeutic tool, eventually finding its way into the armamentarium of plasmapheresis so that we can decrease the number of donors necessary for the manufacturer of factor VIII concentrates. Danazole, a hormone, has also been described as having the ability to elevate factor VIII levels. At the present time it is too early to determine its future role in hemophilia therapy.

Hemophilia, from its early descriptions until the 1960s, was a devasting disorder. With the advent of fractions and comprehensive care the disease has been markedly altered, life span has been increased, and the quality of life improved. As with all other treatment modalities, with time we are beginning to recognize the risks of therapy. Newer technology will clearly afford us the opportunity to remove many of these complications.

General References

Aledort LM (ed) (1975) Recent advances in hemophilia. Ann NY Acad Sci 240: 1–426

Aledort LM (1982) Current concepts in diagnosis and management of hemophilia. Hosp Pract 17: 77–92

Aledort LM (1983) AIDS: an update. Hosp Pract 18: 159–167

Aledort LM, Cohen M, Hilgartner MW, Lipton R (1984) Treatment of hemophiliacs with inhibitors: cost and effect on blood resources. In: Hoyer L (ed) Factor VIII inhibitors. Alan R Liss, New York, pp 253–366

Brinkhous KM, Hemker HC (eds) (1975) Handbook of hemophilia, parts I & II. Elsevier, New York, pp 1–927

Fratantoni J, Aronson D (eds) (1976) Proceedings of a workshop on unsolved therapeutic problems in hemophilia, Bethesda, Md, pp 9–14

Gilbert M, Aledort LM (eds) (1977) Comprehensive care in hemophilia: A team approach. Mt Sinai J Med (NY) 44: 313–479

Hilgartner M (ed) (1982) Hemophilia in the child and adult. Masson, New York

Demography
Anders Larsson and Inga Marie Nilsson

As described earlier in this chapter, the advent of specific substitution therapy in the late 1960s substantially improved the prospects for the hemophiliacs. At about the same time laboratory techniques for assaying factor VIII and factor IX improved, making the diagnoses more reliable, especially in mild cases. These events caused profound changes in the prognosis and demography of hemophilic populations all over the world.

A thorough knowledge of the hemophilic population at hand is required to plan and organize comprehensive hemophilia care. But seemingly simple variables such as incidence, prevalence, distribution of different types and severities of hemophilia, life expectancy, and causes of death and are often difficult and tedious to obtain. However, when national surveys are performed regularly, for instance every 10 or 20 years, it is possible not only to obtain an update of the hemophilic population but also to assess the changes occurring since the last census.

Hemophilia in Sweden

Sweden has longstanding traditions of hemophilia care. The first survey of Swedish hemophiliacs was done by Sköld in 1944. His work was updated in 1962 when Ramgren inventoried all diagnosed hemophiliacs in Sweden.

During the last two decades adequate substitution therapy and prophylaxis came into general use and the number of recognized cases increased. We therefore considered it worthwhile to perform a new census in 1980.

The number of known hemophiliacs in Sweden (8.3 million inhabitants) had more than doubled in 20 years and was 564 at the end of 1980. During the same time the general population increased by 11%. The increase of recognized hemophiliacs was most pronounced among the mild cases, who increased in number from 89 to 307, i.e., by 245%. The corresponding figure for severe hemophilia was only 48%.

The discrepancy in increase of severely and mildly affected hemophiliacs caused a shift in the relative proportion of the severe cases in Sweden. In 1980 only 30% of the hemophiliacs were severe whereas the mild cases constituted 54%. A small group in between (16%) were considered moderately affected. The allocation into severity grades was based solely on the factor VIII:C or IX:C activity in plasma. Thus, patients were classified as severe if the activity was less than 1% of that in normal plasma, moderate if the activity was 1%–4%, and mild if the activity was 5%–25%.

Factor VIII concentrates for treatment of patients with hemophilia A have been available in Sweden since 1956. In that year the so-called fraction I–O was described and this preparation was the only one used in Sweden until the mid 1970s, when new "high purity concentrates" appeared. In 1967 the production of fraction I–O was industrialized (AHFKabi, KabiVitrum AB, Sweden) and since the late 1960s the availability of factor concentrates has not been the limiting factor in the treatment of hemophiliacs in Sweden. Coinciding with the improved availability of factor concentrates there was a salient increase in age at death among Swedish hemophiliacs (Fig. 1.1). The average age at death in severe hemophiliacs was about 20 years until 1968. It increased to 50 years during the period 1968–1980. Similar increases were found for moderate and mild hemophilia. For the latter two categories the median age at death in the period 1968–1980 was only 5 years lower than for Swedish males.

This increase in age at death naturally resulted in improved life expectancy for Swedish hemophiliacs (Fig. 1.2). At the beginning of this century severely affected hemophiliacs had a median life expectancy of only 11 years, which increased to 58 years in the period 1969–1980. The increase was less pronounced among moderate and mild hemophiliacs but they had, of course, a better starting point. Mild and moderate hemophiliacs in Sweden had a median life expectancy of 72 years in 1980, only 3 years less than the corresponding age for males in Sweden. The increased longevity also changed the age distribution of the living hemophiliacs. The age histogram for hemophiliacs has gradually approached that of the Swedish males.

The causes of death has also undergone a change during the last two decades. Until 1957 almost all deaths (90%) were caused by hemorrhagic complications but today an increasing proportion are caused by age-related diseases such as ischemic heart diseases and malignancies. Intracranial hemorrhage, however, seems to have retained its position as the most common single cause of death: among Swedish hemophiliacs it caused one-third of all deaths in the period 1957–1980.

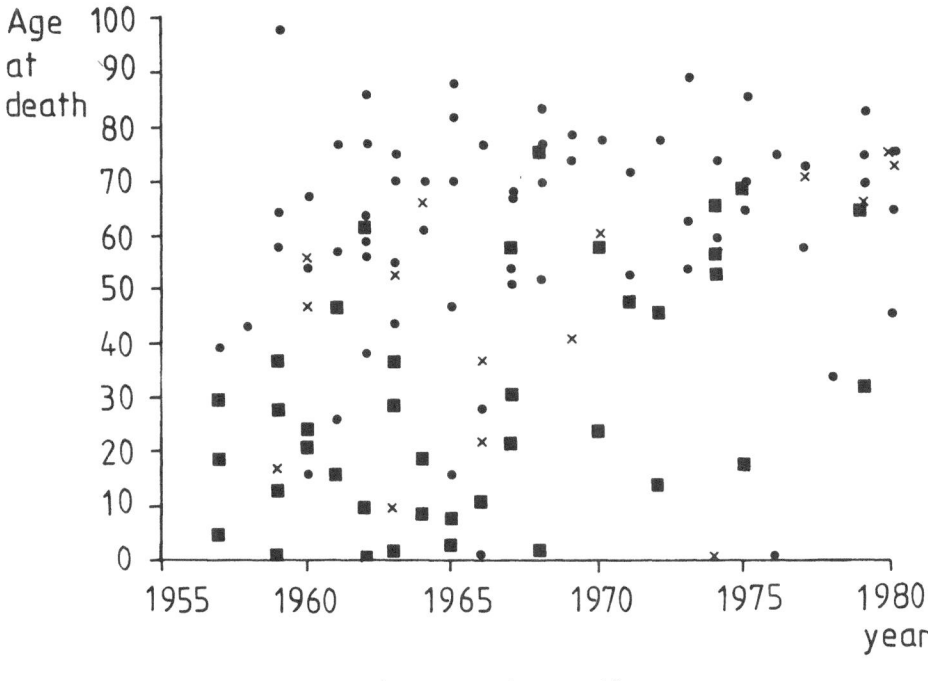

Fig. 1.1. Age at death and severity of hemophilia in Sweden (1957–1980).

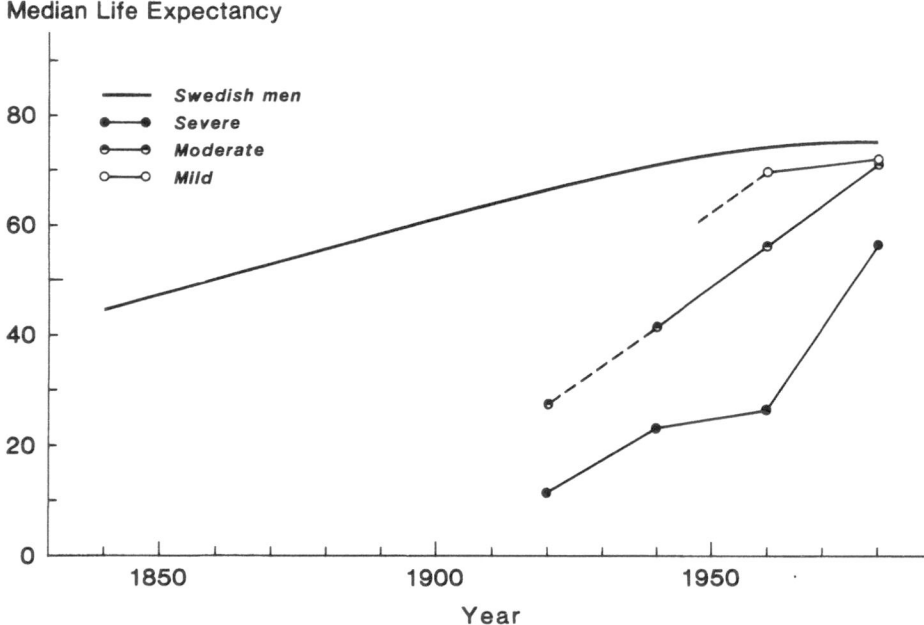

Fig. 1.2. Median life expectancy for severe, moderate, and mild hemophiliacs in Sweden (1831–1980). Corresponding data for Swedish males are given for comparison.

Hemophilia in Other Countries

A number of comprehensive surveys of hemophilia in countries all over the world have been published. Tendencies in demographic changes similar to those found in Sweden have been reported (Tables 1.1, 1.2).

The true incidence and prevalence of hemophilia is not known. Several figures have been suggested, but it seems likely that the prevalence is about 8–11 per 100 000 population. The fact that low figures are reported in several countries might be the result of three factors: genetic differences, low detection rate, and excess mortality. As pointed out previously, the last two are undergoing rapid changes at present. Therefore the global hemophilia population is growing in number and the patients are getting older. With the widespread use of substitution therapy and prophylaxis we shall have an increasing number of older hemophiliacs who will hopefully be less disabled by the bleeding disorder but who will then suffer from other diseases to the same extent as normal men.

Table 1.1. Prevalence of hemophilia in different countries

Country	Hemophiliacs per 100 000 population	Hemophilia A/ hemophilia B	Proportion of severe cases (%)	Reference
U.S.A.	10.0			NHLI 1972[a]
United Kingdom	9.1	85/15	43[b]	Rizza and Spooner 1983
Switzerland	7.0			Koller 1982
Sweden	7.0	81/19	30[e]	Larsson 1984
Finland	6.9[c]			Ikkala et al. 1982
Australia	6.7[d]			Rickard 1976
The Netherlands	6.6	84/16	49[e]	Veltkamp et al. 1974
Canada (Alberta)	6.6	84/16	53[e]	Mant 1980
Norway	6.5	78/22	40[e]	Heger et al. 1980
Austria	6.4[f]			Lechner et al. 1982
Denmark	6.4	80/20	50	Brandt 1979
Scotland (Edinburgh)	6.0			Cash 1976
Belgium	5.8[d,g]			Masure 1976
U.S.A. (Pennsylvania)	5.4	85/15	30[e,h]	Eyster et al. 1980
France	5.3[d]	80/20	71	Allain 1976
Canada (Ontario)	4.9			Hewitt and Milner 1970
Greece	4.6	87/13	77	Mandalaki 1976
West Germany	4.6			Brackman et al. 1976
Japan	3.6	84/16	56[e]	Fukui 1982
Italy	3.5			Mannucci and Ruggeri 1976
Spain	3.3	87/13		Martin-Villar et al. 1976

[a]Quoted by Biggs (1977).
[b]Factor level <2% of normal.
[c]Information in the paper given only for severe hemophilia A. The presented figure is an estimate assuming the proportion of hemophilia A to be 80% and the proportion of severe cases to be 40%.
[d]Estimated prevalence.
[e]Factor level <1% of normal.
[f]Information in the paper only given for hemophiliacs with factor level <3%. The presented figure is an estimate assuming the proportion of hemophiliacs with <3% factor activity to be 50%.
[g]Information in the paper given only for hemophilia A. The presented figure is an estimate assuming the proportion of hemophilia A to be 80%.
[h]43% were moderate cases.

Table 1.2. Age at death

Country	Period	n	Median age at death	Mean age at death	Type, severity	Reference
Denmark	1947–1958	22		25.6	All	Bacher 1980
	1959–1968	23		35.9	All	
	1969–1978	26		41.8	All	
Finland	1930–1939	11		7.8	Severe A	Ikkala et al. 1982
	1950–1959	9		10.2	Severe A	
	1970–1979	6		25.2	Severe A	

continued overleaf

Table 1.2. Age at death

Country	Period	n	Median age at death	Mean age at death	Type, severity	Reference
Global compilation	1975	206	26	29	Mainly severe and moderate	Aledort 1976
Japan	1940–1965	55	6	13.7	A only	Yoshida 1968
	1975–1980	102	16	20.3	A only	Fukui 1982
	1940–1965	16	12.5	15.3	B only	
	1975–1980	23	19	17.8	B only	
Sweden	1957–1968	27	19	23.0	Severe A and B	Larsson 1984
	1969–1980	12	50.5	45.8	Severe A and B	
	1957–1968	39	61	58.6	Mild A and B	
	1969–1980	25	70	66.0	Mild A and B	
U.K.	1969–1974	62		42.3	A only	Biggs 1977
	1976–1980	89		46.7	A only	Rizza and Spooner 1983
	1969–1974	9		33.6	B only	
	1976–1980	18		48.3	B only	
U.S.A.			11.5			NHLI 1972[a]
U.S.A. (Pennsylvania and Virginia	1956–1965	20		34.4	All	Lewis et al. 1976
	1966–1975	21		39.1	All	
U.S.A. (Portland and Oregon)	1910–1930	?		21	?	Stafford et al. 1980
	1970s	?		34	?	

[a] Quoted by Aledort (1976)

References

Aledort LM (1976) The cause of death in hemophiliacs. DHEW Publication No (NIH) 77–1089, pp 9–14

Allain JP (1976) Management of hemophilia in France. Thromb Haemost 35: 553–558

Bacher T (1980) Mortality among patients with haemophilia in Denmark during the period 1949–1978. Ugeskr Laeger 142: 1600–1603

Biggs R (1977) Haemophilia treatment in the United Kingdom from 1969 to 1974. Br J Haematol 35: 487–504

Brackmann HH, Hofmann P, Etzel F, Egli H (1976) Home care of hemophilia in West Germany. Thromb Haemost 35: 544–552

Brandt NJ (1979) Organisation af forebyggelse og behandling. Ugeskr Laeger 141: 1300–1301

Cash JD (1976) International forum: Can a national all voluntary blood transfusion service by adequate blood component therapy cover actual and future needs of AHF? Vox Sang 31: 299–301

Eyster ME, Lewis JH, Shapiro SS, Gill F, Kajani M, Prager D, Djerassi I, Rice S, Lusch C, Keller A (1980) The Pennsylvania hemophilia program 1973–1978. Am J Hematol 9: 277–286

Fukui H (1982) Statistical approach to incidence of hemophilia in Japan. Proc 3rd Int Symp Hemophilia Treatm, Tokyo, pp 31–43

Heger H, Hjort PF, Evensen SA (1980) Helseekonomisk analyse av blödersykdommen i Norge. Tidsskr Nor Laegeforen 100: 948–953

Hewitt D, Milner J (1970) Prevalence of hemophilia in Ontario, 1966. Canad Med Ass J 102: 174–177

Ikkala E, Helske T, Myllylä G, Nevanlinna HR, Pitkänen P, Rasi V (1982) Changes in the life expectancy of patients with severe haemophilia A in Finland in 1930–79. Br J Haematol 52: 7–12

Koller F (1982) The present situation of home care for hemophiliacs in Switzerland. Proc 3rd Int Symp Haemophilia Treatm, Tokyo, pp 187–190

Larsson SA (1984) Hemophilia in Sweden. Studies on demography of hemophilia and surgery in hemophilia and von Willebrand's disease. Acta Med Scand (Suppl) 684

Lechner K, Fasching I, Niessner H, Nowotny C (1982) Current situation of home care in Austria. Proc 3rd Int Symp Hemophilia Treatm, Tokyo, pp 205–213

Lewis JH, Spero JA, Hasiba U (1976) Death in hemophiliacs. JAMA 236: 1238–1239

Mandalaki T (1976) Management of haemophilia in Greece. Thromb Haemost 35: 522–530

Mannucci PM, Ruggeri ZM (1976) Hemophilia care in Italy. Thromb Haemost 35: 531–536

Mant MJ (1980) Congenital coagulation disorders in northern Alberta and surrounding areas of Canada. Clin Invest Med 3: 213–219

Martin-Villar J, Ortega F, Magallon M (1976) Management of hemophilia in Spain. Thromb Haemost 35: 537–543

Masure R (1976) International forum: Can a national all voluntary blood transfusion service by adequate blood component therapy cover actual and future needs of AHF? Vox Sang 31: 309–312

Rickard KA (1976) Haemophilia in Australia. Thromb Haemost 35: 566–569

Rizza CR, Spooner RJD (1983) Treatment of haemophilia and related disorders in Britain and Northern Ireland during 1976–80: Report on behalf of the directors of haemophilia centres in the United Kingdom. Br Med J 286: 929–933

Stafford RS, Hegewald M, Haag C, Wolff L, Lovrien E (1980) Life expectancy in hemophilia. Clin Res 28: 103A

Veltkamp JJ, Schrijver, G, Willeumier W, van de Putte B, van Dijck H (1974) Hemophilia in Netherlands. Results of a survey on the medical, genetic and social situation of the Dutch hemophiliacs. Acta Med Scand (Suppl) 572

Yoshida K (1968) Hemophilia in Japan. Acta Haematol Jpn 31: 5–14

Chapter 2
Diagnostic Imaging Modalities

Until some 20 years ago, radiologic examination meant plain film radiography, with the occasional addition of tomography, or conventional radiography with contrast medium—angiography, myelography, arthrography, intravenous urography, and barium examination of the gastrointestinal tract. During the last 20 years technologic developments of utmost importance have taken place. There have been refinements of conventional radiologic examination, with the addition of low kilovoltage radiography and xeroradiography. The introduction of ultrasonography and computed tomography (CT) has allowed a revolution in the diagnostic workup of many conditions. The information provided by scintimetry using radioactive isotopes also has improved considerably, mainly due to the explosive development of computer technique. Finally, magnetic resonance imaging (MRI), still in its infancy, provides a new dimension in the diagnostic arsenal.

The technical developments have been very rapid, and the vast number of modalities available has totally changed the working conditions for the radiologist. As several of the modalities are not based on roentgen radiation, the term "*diagnostic imaging*" has been settled as a name covering all imaging modalities used in the diagnostic workup of today. Below, the nature of the different modalities will be discussed briefly, as will their diagnostic possibilities and limitations.

Conventional Radiography

The roentgen radiation used for diagnostic purposes is an electromagnetic, ionizing radiation that can penetrate material. The penetration is dependent on the density and thickness of the material penetrated and the wavelength and frequency of the radiation. If a high voltage is used in the generation of the radiation, the penetrating potential will be high, while a low voltage generates radiation with a low penetrating potential. Only a small part of the radiation passes through the material that is radiated, and the pattern of radiation after passage through an object (for instance a human body) may be detected on photographic film, producing a picture. However, modern photographic film has a low sensitivity for roentgen radiation, and therefore screens covered with fluorescing material are used, transferring the radiation pattern to the photographic film. This is *plain film radiography*. Using modern film screen combinations, high spatial resolution (fine details in the pictures) is obtained with low radiation exposure. Such plain film examination gives most information necessary in the evaluation of the skeletal involvement in hemophilic arthropathy, and for survey examination of the thorax and abdomen.

In the evaluation of abdominal lesions, *barium or double contrast (air and barium) examination* of the bowel will change the absorption of radiation passing the abdomen and add important information about lesions of the bowel.

Angiography, using conventional radiography after direct introduction of contrast medium into the arteries, may give information on structural changes of the vessels, but also on lesions that influence the vessel wall or the location and distribution of the vessels. Today angiography has little importance in the diagnostic workup of hemophilic problems, except for presurgical evaluation of pseudotumors (Thomas and Walters 1977).

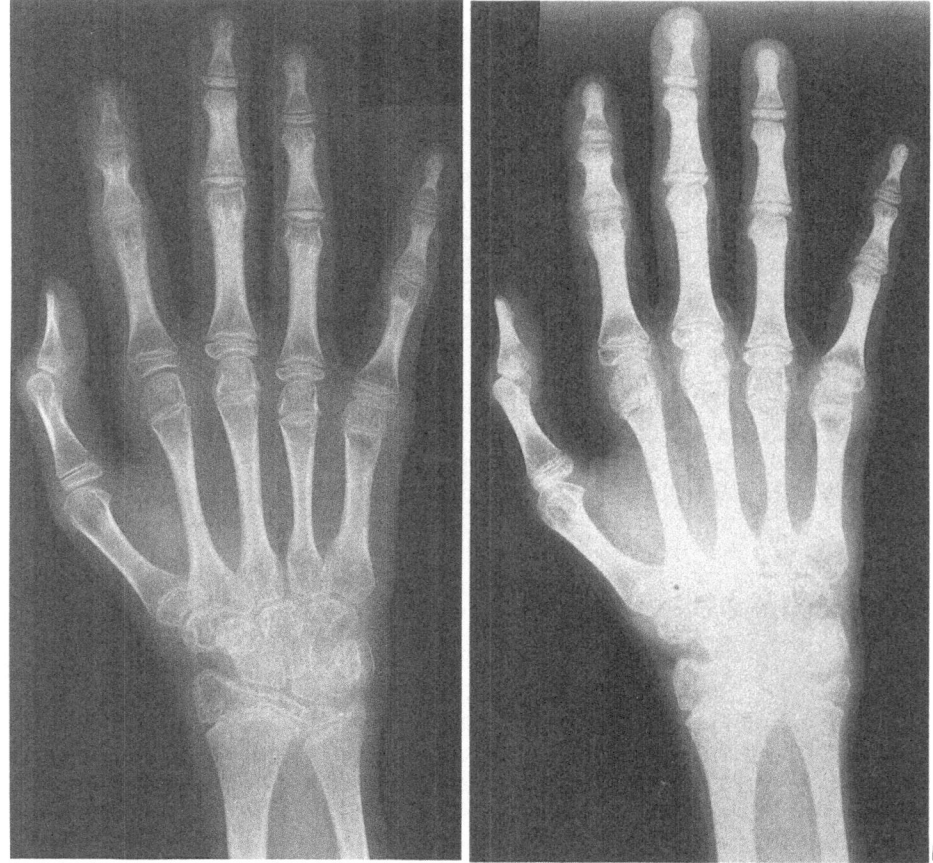

a   b

Fig. 2.1a,b. Comparison of conventional radiography with the low kV technique. **a** On conventional examination of the hand there is detailed information on the skeleton, while the contrast differences between the soft tissue structures are faint. **b** Same occasion, low kV technique. The soft tissues are now well delineated, and differentiation between fat, skin, subcutaneous tissue, muscles, and joint capsules is well defined.

In *intravenous urography*, contrast medium is injected intravenously and excreted by the kidneys, providing information on the kidney, ureters, and bladder, but also secondarily on neighboring structures.

After direct puncture and contrast medium injection in the joint and intraspinal subarachnoid space, respectively, *arthrography* and *myelography* may give important information on intra-articular or intraspinal lesions. *Fistulography* is used for assessing the extent of fistula systems and abscesses.

During the last 10–15 years the *low kilovoltage (kV) technique* has been available also for examination of soft tissue around the joints. The soft tissues have a low absorption potential, and with conventional examination of the skeleton there are no or very faint contrast differences between the soft tissue structures (Fig. 2.1a). Using low kV (25–30 kV) the soft tissues will be well delineated, allowing differentiation between fat, muscle, and tendons (Fig. 2.1b), and effusion within or cyst formation around the joint is easily seen. This low kV technique has proved of great use in the examination of arthritis, and will also give information on the early changes of hemophilic arthropathy.

Xeroradiography

Xeroradiography is an electrostatic imaging system in which selenium is used as a photoconductor. It is a radiographic application of the xerographic process as first described by Carlsson in 1937 (Genant 1981). Xeroradiography has two characteristic features: the phenomenon of edge enhancement and a broad latitude. This means that borders between areas with different absorption potentials for the roentgen radiation are sharply demarcated, even if the difference in absorption between the areas is very slight. It also means that the details of structures with a high density, such as bone, and low density, such as soft tissue and fat, are all well delineated in one and the same image, which is not possible with plain film examination (Fig. 2.2). The largest clinical application for xeroradiography has been in the areas of mammography (Martin 1973; Wolfe et al. 1971). It has also been described for evaluation of soft tissue masses, and for arthritis and metabolic bone disease (Wolfe 1969). It has been tried in hemophilic arthropathy (Ruffato et al. 1979) and has proven especially useful in the early stages, when the changes are confined to the soft tissue. However, the radiation dose is considerably higher than for modern film screen combinations, and there has been no widespread use for xeroradiography in hemophilic patients.

Computed Tomography

With computed tomography (CT) examination thin sections of the body are analyzed separately. The roentgen radiation is given as a fan-beam and the radiation that passes through the body is recorded by xenon or other detectors. During the exposure, the fan-beam and the detectors circulate around the body, and during this rotation a large number of short exposures are performed, often one exposure

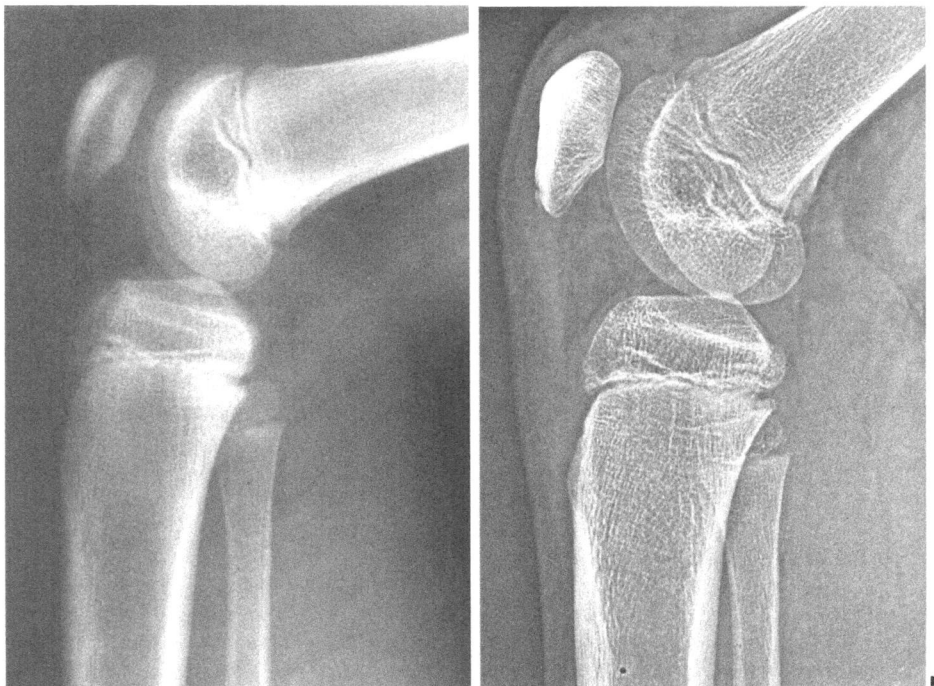

a   b

Fig. 2.2. Comparison of **a** conventional radiography with **b** xeroradiography. With the xeroradiographic technique the borders between structures with different absorption potential are sharply demarcated.

for each degree of rotation. Following the exposure, the measurements recorded by the detectors are registered by a computer, together with information on the beam direction. In a few seconds the computer calculates the radiation attenuation in each point that has been measured in the radiated slice. The size of this point varies but averages about 1 × 1 mm. CT examination gives very good information on structures with small differences in attenuation, while the spatial resolution is less than that obtained at plain film radiography. As the system gives digital information on the attenuation values, it is possible to vary the density level ("window level") and width ("window width") on the screen, and thus from the same image get detailed information on contrast differences both in areas with low and in areas with high attenuation (Fig. 2.3). The amount of attenuation in different areas of the examined slice may be measured and is expressed in Hounsfield Units (HU). As the attenuation values for different tissues are known, the composition of a structure may be analyzed. The computer also allows reconstruction of the measurements, giving images in the frontal, sagittal, or any other plane of the part of the body examined, allowing a three-dimensional evaluation.

Computed tomography has proven invaluable in the assessment of pseudotumors and intracranial or intraspinal hemorrhage. It clearly defines the extent of soft tissue and intramuscular bleeding. It has also has proven to be of great value in the examination of thoracic and abdominal hemorrhages, as will be described in the following chapters.

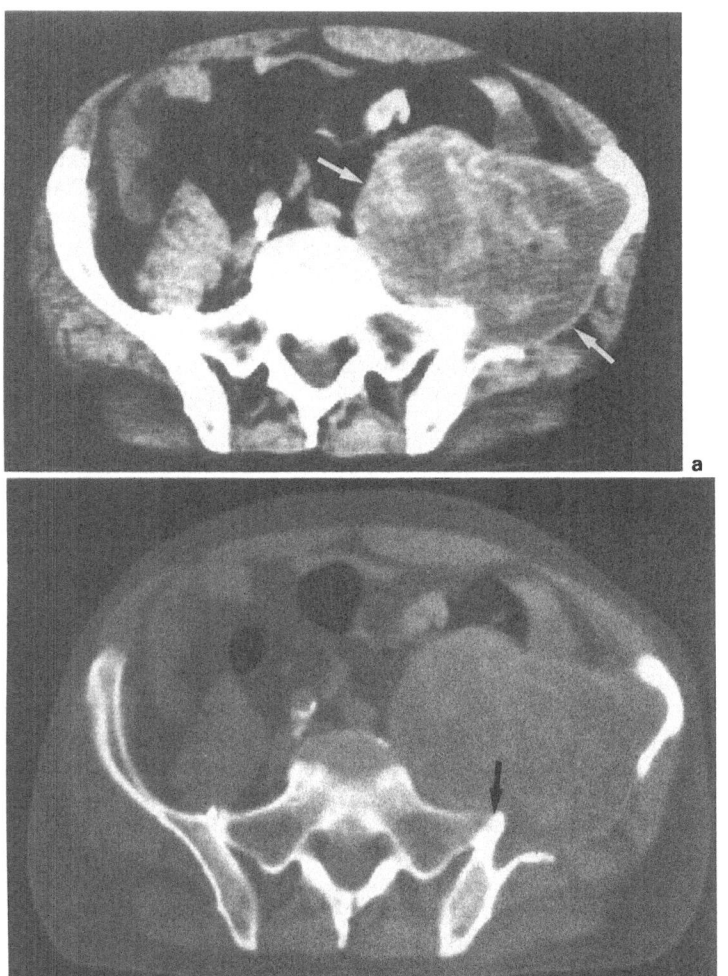

Fig. 2.3a,b. Computed tomography of pelvis with large hemophilic pseudotumor. Different information obtained from the same image. **a** At a low window level and width, the soft tissues, including the pseudotumor with its capsule (*arrows*), and areas of different attenuation within the tumor are well visualized. **b** At a high window level and width, the soft tissue lesions are less visible, while details of the skeleton are distinct, revealing an intact sacroiliac joint (*arrow*).

Scintimetry

In scintimetric examination, radioactive isotopes are injected and the distribution of radioactivity in the body is detected. The information provided by the detection may be digital and transformed to images. The choice of isotope, the compound to which it is bound, and the examination technique differ with the organ system that is to be examined.

For examination of the skeleton, Tc^{99m} is most often used. Nuclear medicine evaluation of bone disease should be carried out using a three-phase study. The first phase is the radionuclide angiogram of the affected area. The second would be immediate images ("blood pool") and the third, delayed bone images with high information density. These images are best recorded via a computer, where the final hard copy can be set up to emphasize either low photon flux in the long bones or the growth zones or both, without reimaging the patient. Both frontal and lateral views of joints such as elbows, knees, and ankles are essential for optimum assessment. In small children converging collimation is an extremely valuable adjunct to magnify the images to obtain better resolution of the involved areas.

Before the era of CT, brain scintimetry was used in the diagnosis of intracranial hemorrhage (Couwan and Mainard 1974). Scintimetry has also been tried for evaluation of hemophilic arthropathy (Cambouroglou et al. 1976; Forbes et al. 1972, 1975). However, today its role in the evaluation of hemorragic complications is small.

Ultrasonography

In the ultrasonographic examination sonic waves with a frequency between 2 and 10 MHz are used. Through a transducer the ultrasound pulses are sent discontinuously. When the pulses reach an area with different acoustic impedance, a small part of the energy is reflected back, and these reflected pulses are transformed to electric energy. These electric impulses are visualized on a TV screen, and repeated sending and receiving of a large number of ultrasound pulses forms a picture that represents a very thin slice of the tissue examined. Being a safe and accurate diagnostic method that provides no radiation hazards and no other known harmful effects, ultrasonography has been established as an important diagnostic tool in a wide range of situations. In hemophilic patients it has proven of value mainly in the diagnosis and follow-up of intramuscular bleeding (Forbes et al. 1977; Aspelin et al. 1984). It has proven of limited value in the evaluation of hemophilic arthropathy. It is sometimes important, but clinically difficult to differentiate synovial swelling from effusion; using modern machines with high frequency and good penetration such differentiation may become possible. The liver, spleen, and retroperitoneal structures, including the kidneys, are well suited for ultrasonographic examination. Because of the poor penetration of air by the ultrasound waves, examination of the chest and the gastrointestinal tract is of limited value.

Magnetic Resonance Imaging

Magnetic resonance imaging (MRI) is founded on the phenomenon of nuclear magnetic resonance, known since the 1940s. If the nuclei of atoms of certain elements are situated in a static magnetic field, they align in the direction of that field. If a radiofrequency field is added in a plane perpendicular to this direction, some nuclei will jump from a low to a high energy state. When the radiofrequency field is withdrawn, the excited nuclei gradually return to the lower energy state and the excess energy is emitted as electromagnetic radiation that may be detected by special sensitive equipment. Recently, methods have been developed not only to record the presence and the relative quantities of the nuclei of these elements in tissues, but also to determine their location in the tissue examined.

Using computer programs for reconstruction that are principally the same as those used for CT, an image of any section of the body may be obtained. This imaging has the potential not only to reveal the anatomy but also to give biochemical tissue characterization, which provides a totally new dimension to diagnostic imaging. However, some problems regarding the examination technique and diagnostic interpretation are still unsolved, and further research is needed to establish MRI as a routine diagnostic modality.

Exciting and promising results on imaging of the normal and pathologic anatomy of the central nervous system, the thorax, and the abdomen have been published (Alfidi et al. 1982; Crooks et al. 1982; Yung et al. 1982). There are also recent reports on musculoskeletal applications of nuclear magnetic resonance (Moon et al. 1983). Very little is known about the MRI appearance of hemorrhagic complications in hemophilia, but the method has a promising potential for examination of the central nervous system and the thoracic and abdominal cavities. It might also give information on structural and biochemical changes in the early development of hemophilic arthropathy and soft tissue bleeding.

Possible Complications Caused by the Examinations

Several of the diagnostic imaging modalities discussed above (conventional radiography, xeroradiography, CT, and scintimetry) expose the patient to a dose of ionizing radiation. The potential damage caused by high dosages of ionizing radiation is well known, e.g., cancer, leukemia, fetal injuries, etc. The dosages given with the examinations discussed in this chapter are very small, and the risk for the individual patient is diminutive but not negligible. For this reason the International Committee for Radiation Protection (I.C.R.P.) has recommended that the dose given in every situation should be held as low as possible. This should be borne in mind when dealing with a patient group like hemophiliacs, as the injury caused by the radiation is additive and during their lifetime they will be examined several times.

Until now there has been no biologic hazard reported with ultrasonography, and it should therefore be the method of choice when possible, especially in examination of soft tissue bleedings. Magnetic resonance imaging has proven to be biologically safe so far, and in the future may replace some of the modalities using ionizing radiation.

Most of the methods are noninvasive, providing no risks to patients other than the radiation. However, angiography, myelography, and arthrography involve puncture of an artery, the spinal canal, and a joint, respectively. In hemophilia serious bleeding is possible after such punctures. However, with adequate replacement therapy before examination there should be little or no extra risk and during the last 10 years no serious bleeding complications following these examinations have been reported.

References

Alfidi RJ, Haaga JR, El Yoused SJ, Bryan PJ, Fletcher BD, Lipuma JP, Morrison SC, Kaufman B, Richey JB, Hinshaw WS, Kramer DM, Yeung HN, Cohen AM, Butler HE, Ament AE, Lieberman JM (1982) Preliminary experimental results in humans and animals with a superconducting, whole-body, nuclear magnetic resonance scanner. Radiology 143: 175–181

Aspelin P, Pettersson H, Sigurjonson S, Nilsson IM (1984) Ultrasonographic examination of muscle hematomas in hemophiliacs. Acta Radiol 25: 513–516

Cambouroglou G, Papathanassiou B, Koutoulidis C, Bossinakou I, Mandalaki T (1976) Haemophilic arthropathy surveyed with whole-body gamma-camera scintigraphy. Acta Orthop Scand 47: 607–612

Couwan RJ, Mainard CD (1974) Trauma to the brain and extracranial structures. Semin Nucl Med 4: 319–338

Crooks LE, Mills CM, Davis PL, Brandt-Zawaszki M, Hoenninger J, Arakana M, Watts J, Kaufman L (1982) Visualization of cerebral and vascular abnormalities by NMR imaging. The effects of imaging parameters on contrast. Radiology 144: 843–852

Forbes CD, Greig WR, Prentice CRM, McNicol GP (1972) Radioisotope knee joint scans in haemophilia and Christmas disease. J Bone Joint Surg [Br] 54: 468–475

Forbes DC, James W, Prentice CRM, Greig W (1975) A comparison of thermography, radioisotope scanning and clinical assessment of the knee joints in haemophilia. Clin Radiol 26: 41–45

Forbes CD, Lowe GDU, Prentice CRM (1977) Ultrasonography in hemophilia. Lancet I: 1064–1065

Genant HK (1981) Xeroradiography. In: Resnick D and Niwayama G (eds) Diagnosis of bone and joint disorders, vol 1. Saunders, Philadelphia London Toronto, pp 374–379

Martin JE (1973) Xeromammography—an improved diagnostic method. A review of 250 biopsied cases. AJR 117: 90–94

Moon KL Jr, Genant HK, Helms CA, Chafetz NI, Crooks LE, Kaufman L (1983) Musculoskeletal applications of nuclear magnetic resonance. Radiology 147: 161–171

Ruffato C, Pedoja G, Traldi A (1979) Xeroradiographic study of haemophilic arthropathy. Diagn Imaging 48: 103–112

Thomas ML, Walters HL (1977) The angiographic findings in a hemophilic pseudotumor of bone. Australas Radiol 21: 346–349

Wolfe JN (1969) Xeroradiography of the bones, joints and soft tissues. Radiology 93: 583–587

Wolfe JN, Dooley R, Harkins LE (1971) Xeroradiography of the breast: A comparative study with conventional mammography. Cancer 28: 1569–1571

Yung IR, Bailes DR, Burl M (1982) Initial clinical evaluation of a whole-body nuclear magnetic resonance (NMR) tomography. J Comput Assist Tomogr 6: 1–18

Chapter 3

Hemophilic Arthropathy

As mentioned in Chap. 1, references to a bleeding disorder that affected primarily males appeared in ancient writings (Rosner 1969) but it was not until the nineteenth century that Otto (1803) and Legg (1872) reported that hemophilia was frequently associated with an arthritic diathesis. Several papers mistakenly speculated on the reason for the increased incidence of rheumatism, gouty arthritis, or tuberculous arthritis. Volkmann (1868) first stated that in hemophilia, hemarthroses could occur spontaneously or due to an insignificant cause. In 1892, König demonstrated that these arthropathies were secondary to intra-articular bleeding. He gave a detailed description of the clinical findings which remains valid to the present time. A lack of hemotologic treatment led him to suggest that mild compression and immobilization was the recommended treatment for these hemarthroses.

Clinical Considerations

Orthopedic care for the hemophiliac did not advance through the first half of the twentieth century until Jordan (1958), in his classic treatise *Hemophilic Arthropathies*, devised a system of bracing and cast correction for the musculoskeletal manifestations of hemophilia. With the advent of factor replacement therapy for these patients, his methods were rapidly outdated as physiotherapy and surgery became the mainstays of orthopedic treatment. While many problems are still unresolved, the thrust of treatment at present should be prevention of these musculoskeletal complications.

Forrai (1979) has correctly pointed out that "hemophilic arthropathy is a single, long process which starts as an acute intra-articular hemarthrosis and eventually leads to disabling regression through several episodes of bleeding, destruction of cartilage and degenerative changes of the subchondral bony tissues. Its course is slow and progressive, although not without episodes of relative comfort, and there are no specific clinical, patho-morphologic or radiologic stages of the disease. Nevertheless, for practical reasons, some sort of staging becomes necessary to characterize the patient's condition." König divided the destructive process into three stages: (1) the stage of the first bleeding, the hemarthrosis of the bleeder; (2) the inflammatory stage, panarthritis in the bleeder's joints; and (3) the regressive stage, which causes permanent deformity of the bleeder's joints, the contracture of the joints.

DePalma (1967) further divided arthropathy into four grades, and more recently Arnold and Hilgartner (1977) have described five stages in which they attempt to correlate the clinical and radiologic features. However, it has long been our feeling that there is frequently little correlation between the clinical and the radiologic status. Jordan (1958) stated that "it is amazing to see how a marked degree of articular destruction with extensive thinning of cartilage leaving a joint space of only a few millimetres, is compatible with a considerable range of motion." Therefore, a careful clinical and radiologic evaluation of the patient is necessary in order to plan treatment properly for the individual patient. An evaluation that takes into account several clinical and radiologic factors will be presented later in this chapter.

Clinical Course

Almost every severe hemophiliac will experience a hemarthrosis during the first two decades of life and it is rare for him to enter the third decade without some evidence of arthropathy. There is no difference in the clinical manifestations of factor VIII and factor IX deficiencies. van Creveld et al. (1971) pointed out that despite early treatment joint degeneration is progressive, and Lévine (1974) demonstrated that even on home care destruction will continue and new joint involvement is noted. Early treatment has thus modified but not eliminated the musculoskeletal manifestations of this disease.

The first hemarthrosis usually occurs in the first decade and almost any joint in the extremity may be affected. Jordan (1958) and Duthie et al. (1972) suggested that the knees, elbows, and ankles are most commonly involved in decreasing order of frequency. Hip, shoulder, and wrist involvement is less common, and bleeding into the small joints of the hands and feet without significant trauma is rare. Temporomandibular and spine involvement is exceedingly rare. Factor replacement has changed the total as well as the relative frequency of joints involved, as will be discussed below.

No one has adequately explained why certain joints are more commonly involved than others. Jordan proposed, and it has been generally accepted, that trauma precedes all hemarthroses and that "spontaneous hemarthroses" are secondary to microtrauma. It has subsequently been demonstrated that trauma to the synovium is more common in the complex joints, such as the knee and elbow, than it is in the ball and socket joints, such as the hip and shoulder. Because of the large synovial surfaces present within the knee and elbow and because of the rotatory stresses within these joints, synovial trauma is quite common. The frequency of ankle involvement has been attributed to the frequency of external trauma to this joint. These hypotheses, however, must be tempered by the fact that the complex temporomandibular joint is rarely involved and that arthropathy of the fingers is rare despite frequent trauma.

The clinical picture of joint bleeding is characterized by pain, swelling, and limitation of motion. A prodromal period or "aura" has been described as a painless but distinct feeling which the patient appreciates prior to the pain of an acute hemarthrosis (Gilbert 1977). This may be accompanied by mild stiffness and lasts up to 1 h. If left untreated, the joint becomes warm, swollen, and tense. Flexion, limitation of motion, and secondary muscle spasm follow. It has been postulated that bleeding will continue until the intra-articular pressure is raised to that of the bleeding vessel. The clinical course following the first hemarthrosis is variable. In some joints the hemarthrosis will resolve completely, but others will bleed recurrently despite what seems to be adequate treatment. Joints displaying a tendency towards such recurrent bleeding have been termed "target joints" (Aronstam et al. 1979). This corresponds to the second stage described by König. Complete resolution is theoretically possible but more commonly there is persistent synovial thickening, tenderness at the joint line, and moderate limitation of joint motion.

The pain usually responds quickly to factor replacement. If treatment is instituted early, the other objective findings will resolve after several days.

The progression may take one of three courses:

1. With persistent treatment the findings may resolve, usually with some permanent damage. Crepitus and moderate limitation of motion may be associated with some degenerative changes on radiologic examination.

2. On occasion, the inflammatory nature of this irritation will become prominent and a synovial hypertrophy with large effusions which do not respond to transfusion therapy will ensue. This clinical state has been termed "hemophilic synovitis" and will be dealt with in a separate chapter (Chap. 4).

3. Recurrence of the panarthritis will eventually, over a variable, usually prolonged period, lead to the last stage of arthropathy, which is characterized by a painful contracted joint in which bleeding is not a significant problem.

Chronic inflammation with its concomitant hyperemia will cause early appearance of epiphyseal growth centers, epiphyseal overgrowth, and longitudinal overgrowth. The clinical manifestations of longitudinal overgrowth are most obvious at the knee, where the adjacent growth plates contribute almost 70% to the length of the extremity. Kingma (1965) has shown that affected limbs might be 2–3 cm longer in these patients. This only becomes clinically evident after an associated flexion contracture is corrected. Circumferential enlargement of the epiphyseal center is manifest by the "enlarged knee," which is accentuated by the associated muscle atrophy. There may also be premature fusion of the epiphysis to the metaphysis, which can cause shortening and angular deformity (Caffey and Schlesinger 1940); such fusion is not, however, common.

Involvement of Different Joints

As mentioned above, the number of affected joints and the degree of the arthropathy vary greatly with the age of the patient and the severity of the disease, while the type of hemophilia (A or B) does not influence the arthropathy. In severe hemophilia the elbow and knee are most often affected first, and bleeding may occur by age 2–4 years. With increasing age, more joints may be involved, and joint destruction progresses. After the age of 20–25 the incidence of bleeding levels off. Pettersson and Nilsson (1982) have shown that bleeding and ensuing arthropathy may occur into previously unaffected joints even in the older patient.

With modern treatment there has been a revolutionary improvement in the number of joints involved and the degree of destruction. Also, the distribution of involvement of the different joints has changed during the last decades. In a recent investigation (Pettersson and Nilsson 1984), we reviewed the fraction of affected joints in two Swedish hemophilic populations:

Population I consisted of 42 patients with severe hemophilia A, aged 1–25 years, admitted to the International Hemophiliac Treatment and Training Center in Malmö between 1958 and 1962. At that time they had had no specific treatment. All great joints were radiographed at admittance.

Population II consisted of 45 patients with severe hemophilia A, aged 1–25 years, on continuous prophylaxis for up to 18 years. At follow-up examination in 1984 all great joints were radiographed.

Table 3.1 compares the percentage of affected joints in the two populations. In the 1984 examination there was a considerable decrease in the fraction of involved joints except for the ankles, where an increase was noted. This increase has been observed at other Hemophilia Centers as well. It may be explained by the patients' increased ability to practice sports and more active games, as the other joints are preserved and the total health situation has so dramatically improved due to modern treatment.

Table 3.1. Comparison of joint involvement in 42 severe hemophiliacs aged 1–25 years, examined between 1958 and 1962 (population I), and 45 other severe hemophiliacs of the same age, on continuous prophylaxis, examined in 1984 (population II)

Joint	Joint involvement (%)	
	Population I	Population II
Shoulder	9	2
Elbow	43	23
Hip	4	0
Knee	55	10
Ankle	31	46

Pathology

It is important to trace the concomitant pathologic changes occurring within the joint. The first and most important pathologic description of the hemophilic joint was published by Swanton in 1959. She followed a series of hemophilic dogs and was able to describe the natural history of the arthropathy. She demonstrated that the primary site of hemorrhage was the synovium and that a discrete hematoma developed which would eventually burst into the joint, allowing bleeding to continue until intra-articular pressure was raised.

The time when bleeding is limited to the synovium probably accounts for the prodromal symptoms or "aura" that the hemophiliac notes before swelling, pain, and spasm. Following resorption of early hemarthrosis, changes are limited to the synovial tissue. Villous hypertrophy is associated with increased vascularity. Phagocytic cells are laden with hemosiderin pigments and perivascular infiltration is noted. Fibrosis of the subsynovial tissue follows. Storti et al. (1969) have described extensive vascular hyperplasia and an "angiomatoid" appearance of the synovium.

These changes are not dissimilar to those seen in pigmented villonodular synovitis, and the radiographic changes in this disorder and hemophilia may be similar. Later in the disease progressive fibrosis of the synovial tissue is noted. This hypertrophic and hyperemic tissue is eventually replaced by fibrosis. This correlates with the progression from König's second to third stage of arthropathy and may account for the decrease in incidence of bleeding in the destroyed joint.

Cartilaginous changes do not occur until after repeated hemarthroses, and early investigators were only able to reproduce the synovial changes by injecting blood into the joints of experimental animals. Key (1932), Soeur (1949), Young and Hudacek (1954), and Wolf and Mankin (1965) were unable to reproduce the cartilaginous and bone changes that were characteristic of hemophilic arthropathy. Finally, in 1967, Hoaglund was able to reproduce these changes in growing puppies. The articular changes that are first noted include microfibrillation, pannus formation on the surface, and metachromatic staining changes. Clumping of chondrocytes and cellular death are followed by microscopic pitting and separation of cartilage fragments from bone. Subchondral osteoporosis is noted (Fig. 3.1). The subchondral cysts that appear are similar to those seen in other arthritides and are synovial lined and nonhemorrhagic.

Three factors can be implicated in the process of cartilage breakdown. These are: (1) enzymatic degradation, (2) a direct effect of iron, and (3) mechanical factors. Proteolytic enzymes have been shown to degrade cartilage (Harris et al. 1970). Hilgartner et al. (1972) demonstrated increased levels of acid phosphatase and cathepsin D. Prostaglandin levels are also elevated (Robinson and Granda, 1974). It is of interest that in the fibrotic or end-stage arthropathy, the levels of cathepsin D are decreased. Ghadially and Roy (1967), Hough et al. (1976), and Duthie and

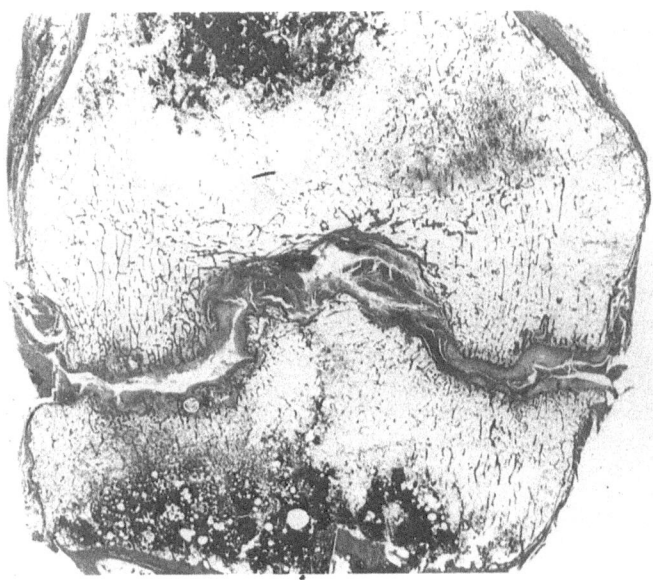

Fig. 3.1. Frontal section of specimen with advanced hemophilic arthropathy. There is fibrillation and irregularity of the articular cartilage of the knee, with subchondral bone irregularity and osteopenia.

Stein (1977) have demonstrated siderosomes within the chondrocytes and have implicated them as a direct cause of cell death and cartilage degradation. In addition, mechanical factors such as increased joint pressure, lack of subchondral support secondary to osteoporosis and cyst formation, immobilization, and interference with normal nutrition must contribute to the joint destruction. Further study is required to determine the relative importance of all these factors.

Diagnostic Imaging

In the diagnostic workup of hemophilic arthropathy, conventional radiography on plain films in most cases is sufficient to provide detailed information on the skeletal destruction of the joint. However, it does not reveal the pathology of the synovium and cartilage. Arthrography and other diagnostic modalities such as CT, ultrasound, scintimetry, and MRI may be used in rare selected cases to give additional information.

Below, hemophilic arthropathy as it appears in conventional radiography will be discussed in detail, and after that the possibilities provided by other diagnostic modalities will be presented briefly.

Conventional Radiography

Together with the pseudotumor, hemophilic arthropathy offers the most characteristic changes from a radiologic point of view. Several of these changes are common to all joints, appearing in a given sequence during the progression of the joint destruction. The lesions caused by the repeated hemarthroses may also give characteristic pathologic patterns in different joints, and thus there are radiologic changes specific for the different joints. Below, the general changes common to all joints will first be discussed, followed by a description of the radiologic changes characteristic for specific joints.

Concerning the examination technique, frontal and lateral views of the joint are sufficient in most cases. However, correct assessment of the knee joint demands that the frontal views be taken with the patient standing, and for the planning of surgical intervention such as osteotomy or arthroplasty special projections are needed, for example to assess the mechanical axis of the leg (Maquet 1976).

For examination of patients with contractures or other malalignments between the articulating bones, the routine AP and lateral views must be modified according to the patient's disability in order to get proper projections of the joint, as already stressed by Jordan (1958). In the knee, it is necessary to get the central beam parallel to the tibial plateau. It should also be stressed that a flexion contracture may mean that the distance between the joint and the radiographic film is large, leading to a magnification that may be misinterpreted as hemophilic epiphyseal enlargement.

General Changes

The radiologic appearance of the initial hemarthrosis is that of distention of the joint. There is an increased soft tissue density, caused by the blood within the joint and the edema of the surrounding tissues. The capsule may be distended and bulge, and the joint space may be widened (Fig. 3.2). It is not uncommon for several bleeding episodes to resolve without causing permanent radiologic changes (Brown et al. 1982), but it has also been shown that two acute hemarthroses may cause persistent synovial hypertrophy with hemosiderin deposition and fibrosis which is visible as increased density in the periarticular soft tissue (Fig. 3.3) (Arnold and Hilgartner 1977; Wood et al. 1969). The density may vary and in some cases may simulate calcifications (Fig. 3.4) (DePalma 1967).

As most intra-articular bleedings occur during childhood, many of the changes seen are the result of persistent hyperemia upon the growing skeleton. As mentioned earlier, the increased blood flow in the periarticular tissues causes accelerated ossification and growth of the epiphyses (Figs. 3.5, 3.6).

Concomitant with the overgrowth is osteopenia, resulting from the combination of hyperemia and disuse of the limb. The former causes a selective epiphyseal osteopenia, with a coarse trabecular pattern (Fig. 3.6) which is similar to that of other chronic childhood arthritides such as juvenile rheumatoid arthritis. The disuse can cause severe generalized osteopenia with thinning of the diaphyseal cortex (see Fig. 3.9).

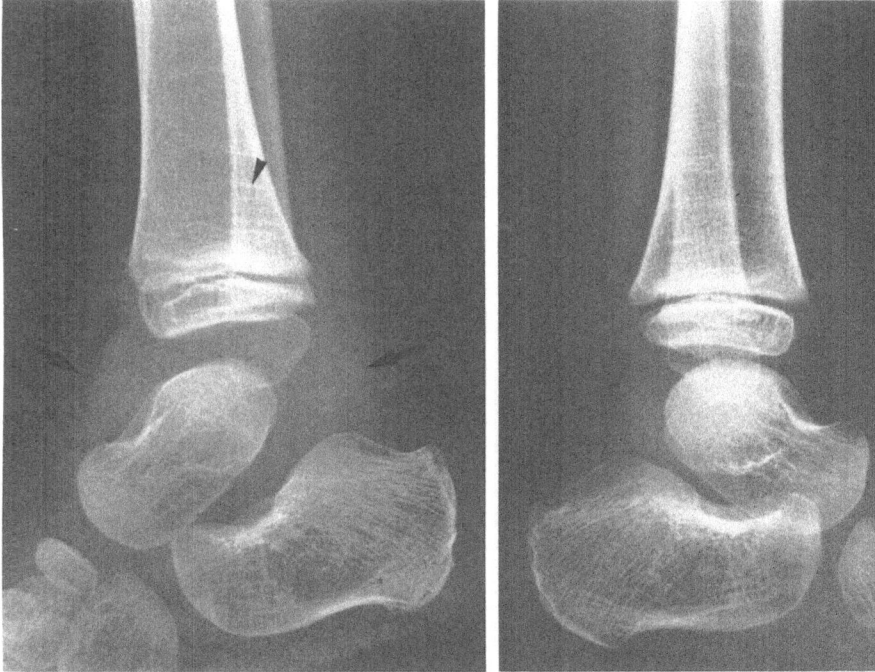

a   b

Fig. 3.2. Comparison of **a** hemarthroses of the ankle and subtalar joint with **b** the normal contralateral joints. 5-year-old with severe hemophilia A. The joint capsule bulges (*arrow*), and the joint spaces are widened between the tibia and talus as well as in the subtalar joints. Note the Harris' lines (*arrowhead*).

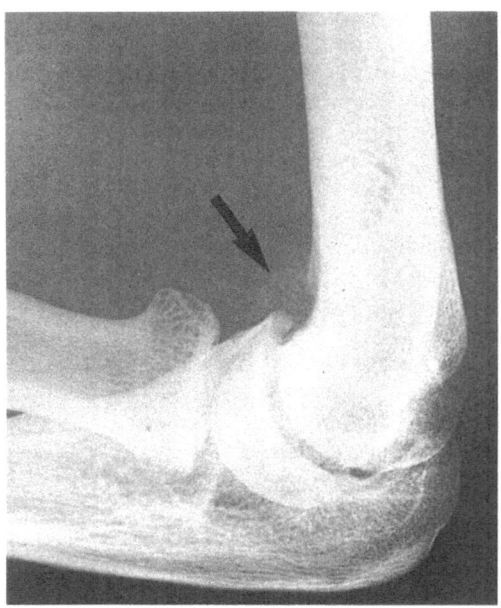

Fig. 3.3.

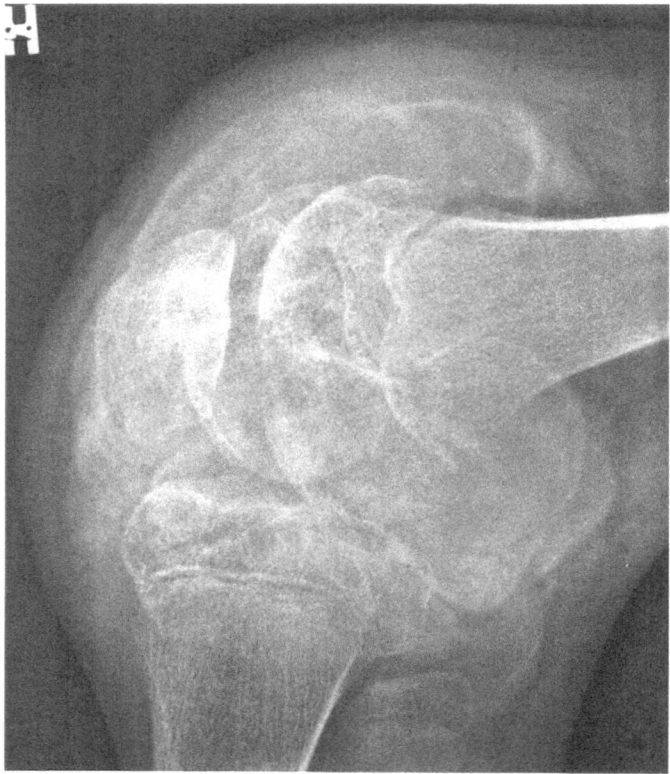

Fig. 3.4.

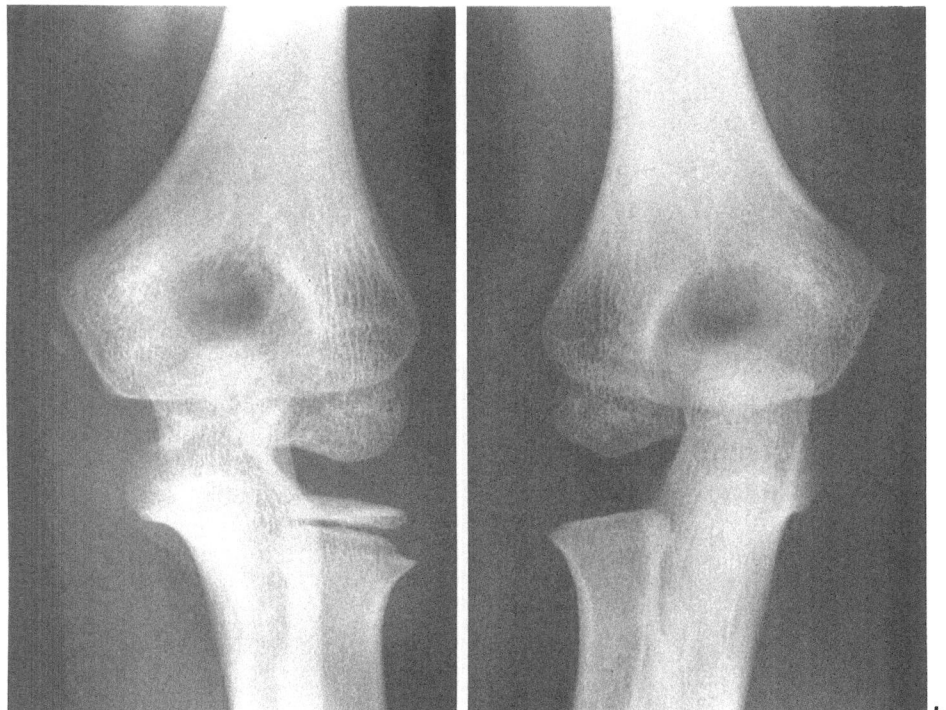

a   b

Fig. 3.5. a Accelerated ossification in the elbow compared with **b** the normal contralateral joint. 7-year-old with severe hemophilia A. Owing to hyperemia in the affected joint, the ossification center of the medial epicondyle has ossified, and the radial head has ossified and enlarged, while none of these centers has ossified on the normal side. The humeral capitellum is larger on the affected side.

Fig. 3.3. Increased periarticular soft tissue density after repeated hemarthroses. 19-year-old with severe hemophilia B. After several hemarthroses there is hypertrophy of the synovia, with hemosiderin deposition and fibrosis (*arrow*).

Fig. 3.4. Pronounced periarticular soft tissue density. 11-year-old with severe hemophilia A. The synovia is hypertrophied and the capsule is distended. The hemosiderin deposition causes a pronounced increase of the density, simulating calcification.

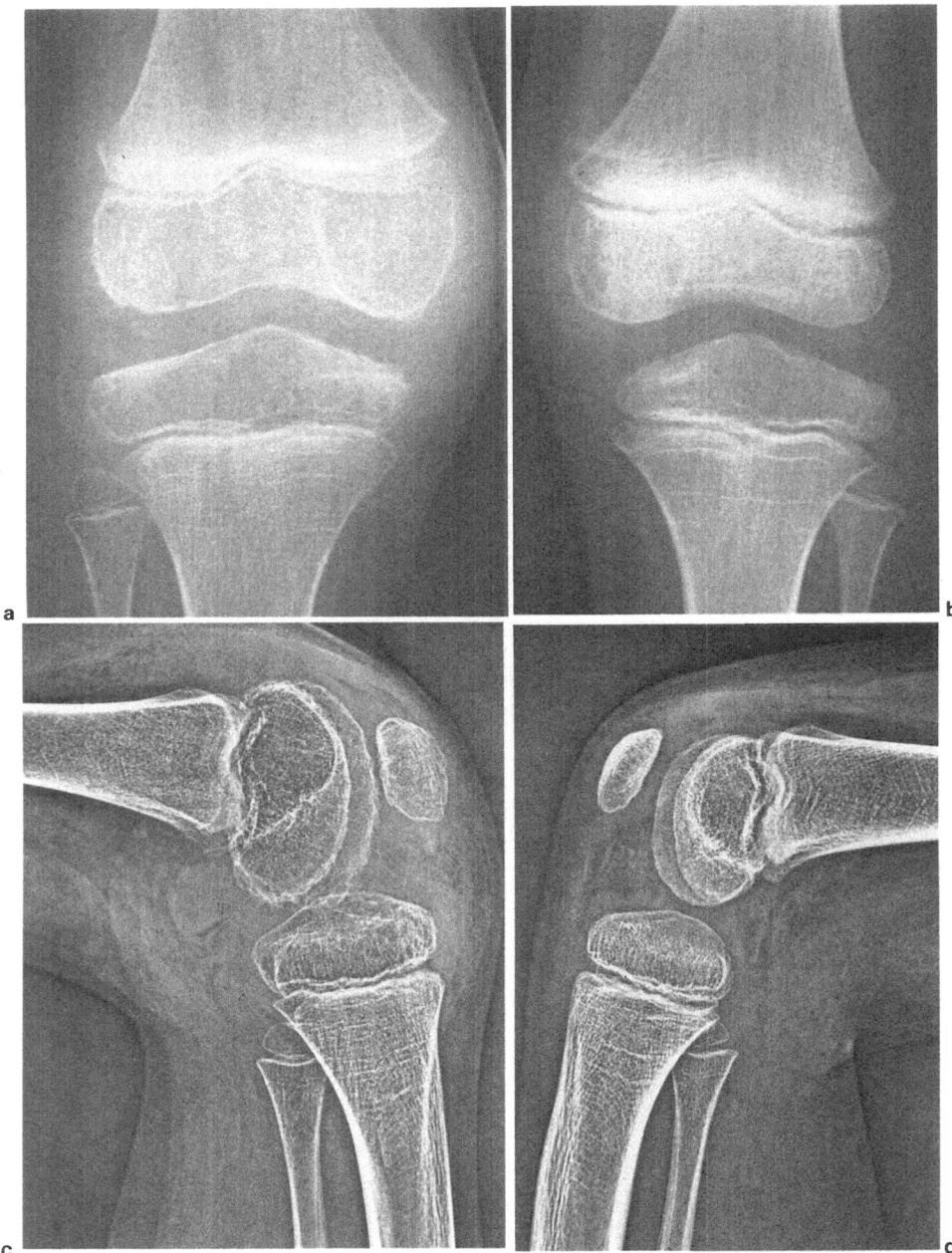

Fig. 3.6a–d. Accelerated growth and osteopenia. 7-year-old with moderate hemophilia A. **a** and **c** the right, affected knee; **b** and **d** the left, normal knee. The frontal views are conventional radiographs, the lateral views xeroradiographs. On the affected side, the femoral, tibial, and fibular epiphyses as well as the patella are increased in size and osteopenic. There is a slight subchondral irregularity. The joint capsule is bulging. Note the Harris' lines, on both sides.

Progressive degeneration of the cartilage results in joint space narrowing and subchondral bone irregularity (Fig. 3.7). Erosions and subchondral cysts appear as the degeneration progresses (Fig. 3.8). The combination of osteopenia and cyst formation can cause subchondral collapse with loss of congruity of the joint surfaces, resulting in displacement and angulation of the bone ends (Fig. 3.9). In this stage, the changes may be similar to, and in fact are, expressions of secondary osteoarthritis (Fig. 3.10). Subchondral sclerosis may be noted but osteophyte formation is rarely severe even in the advanced stages of destruction (Fig. 3.9) (Stoker and Murray 1974).

In the past, when adequate treatment was not available, severe deformity and joint destruction were common. On rare occasions, spontaneous bone ankylosis did occur, especially in the knee and ankle (Fig. 3.11) (Ahlberg 1965; Stoker and Murray 1974).

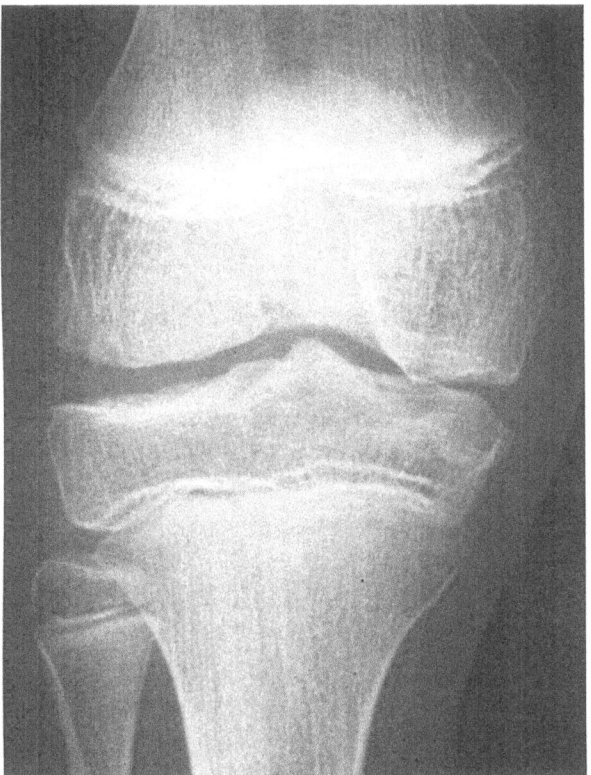

Fig. 3.7. Same patient as in Fig. 3.6, 11 years old. In addition to the increased size of the epiphyses, and the osteopenia with a course trabecular pattern, the joint space is moderately narrowed and the subchondral irregularity is more pronounced.

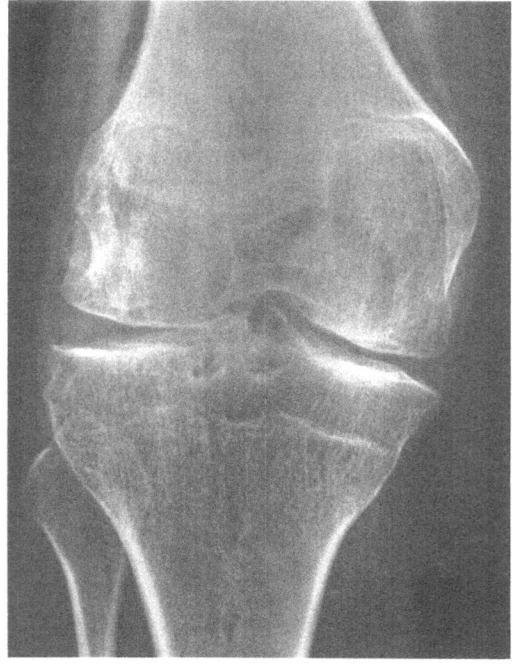

△ Fig. 3.8.   Fig. 3.9. ▽

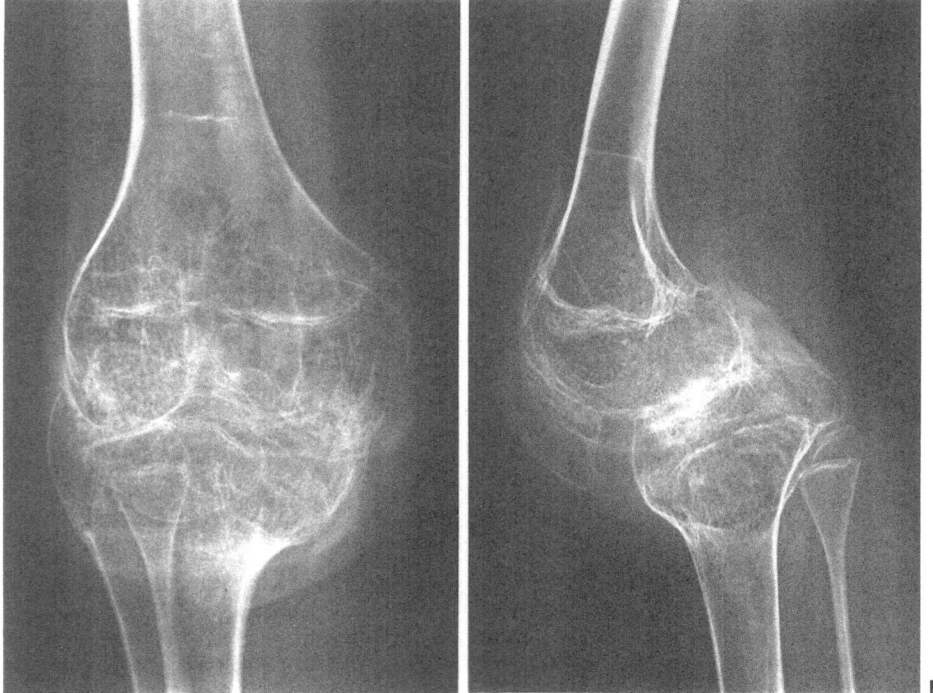

a   b

Fig. 3.8. Same patient as in Figs. 3.6 and 3.7, 23 years old. In addition to the previously described abnormalities, there are now erosions and subchondral cysts. The subchondral bone is slightly sclerotic.

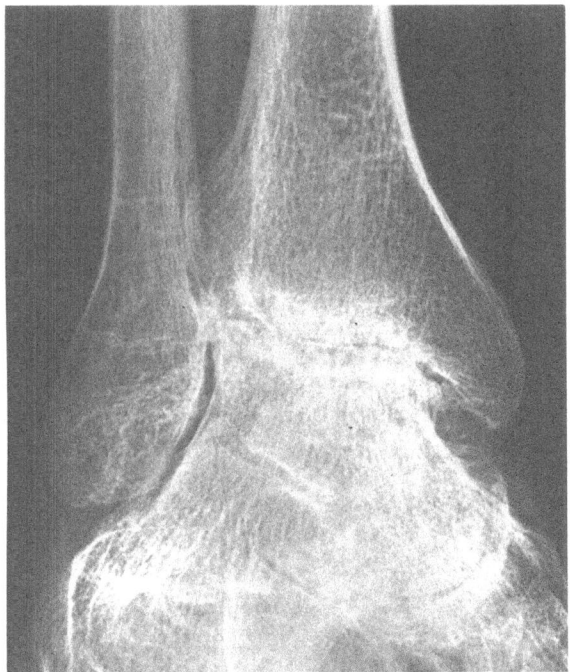

Fig. 3.10. Advanced hemophilic arthropathy. 26-year-old with severe hemophilia A. In this stage the arthropathy is in many respects similar to advanced osteoarthritis.

Growth arrest (Harris') lines (Fig. 3.6), often described as part of the radiologic changes in hemophilic arthropathy (Wood et al. 1969), are totally nonspecific, occurring after periods of severe stress in any growing individual.

The progression of hemophilic arthropathy in the knee, the most commonly involved joint before the era of modern treatment, is illustrated in Fig. 3.12.

Fig. 3.9a,b. Advanced hemophilic arthropathy, knee joint. 15-year-old with severe hemophilia B. **a** frontal and **b** lateral view. There is a pronounced generalized osteopenia. The cartilage is totally destroyed and there is an incongruity between the bone ends, with displacement and severe posterior subluxation of the tibia. In spite of the advanced abnormalities, there is no osteophyte formation.

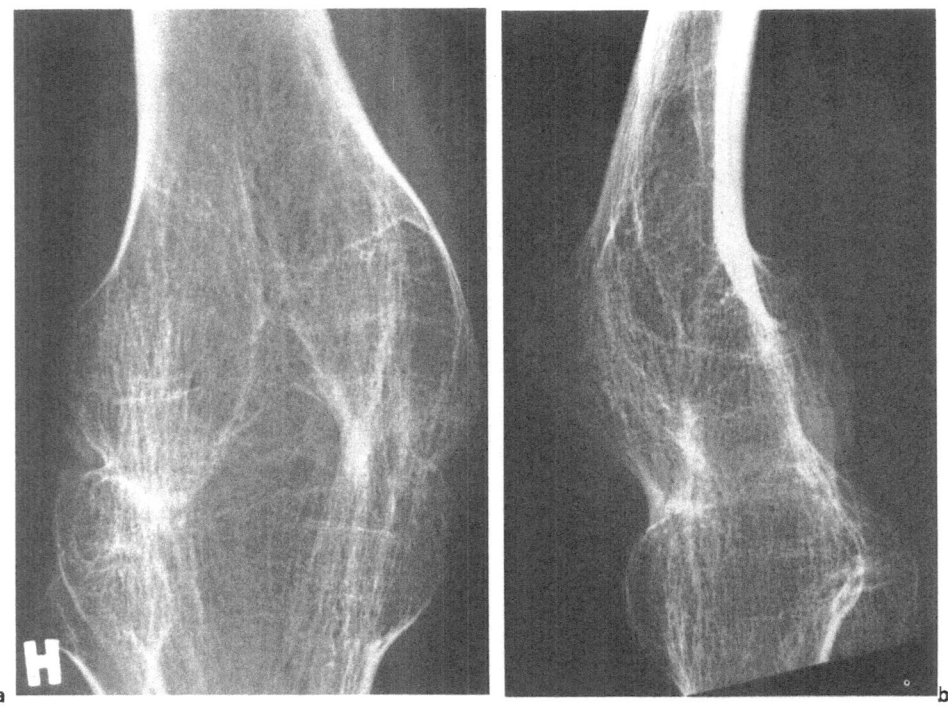

Fig. 3.11a,b. Ankylosis of the knee joint. 33-year-old with severe hemophilia A. Spontaneous ankylosis is rare but may occur especially in the knee and ankle joints.

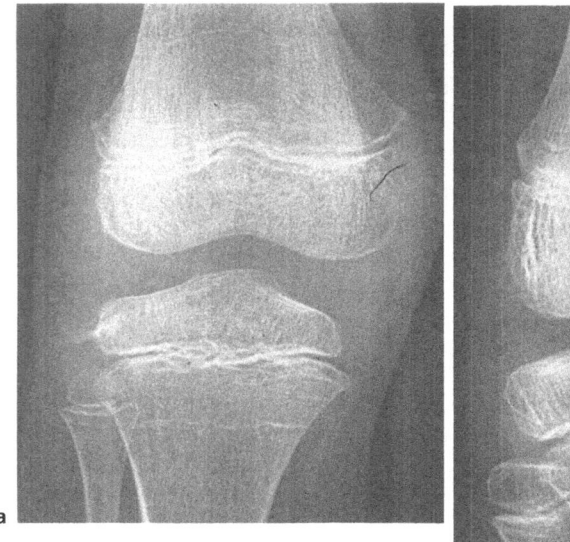

Fig. 3.12.

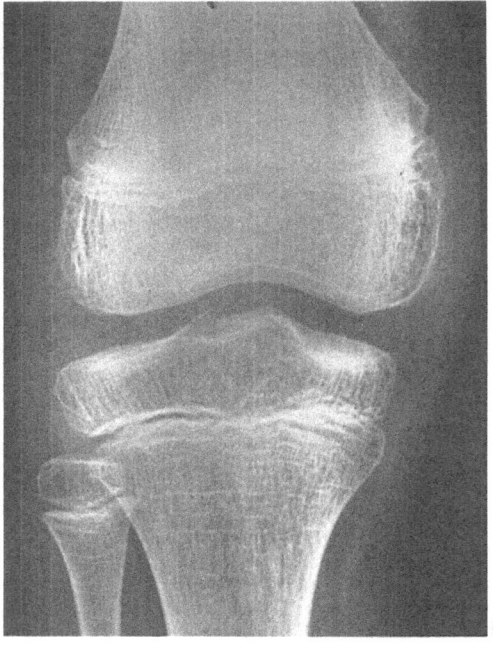

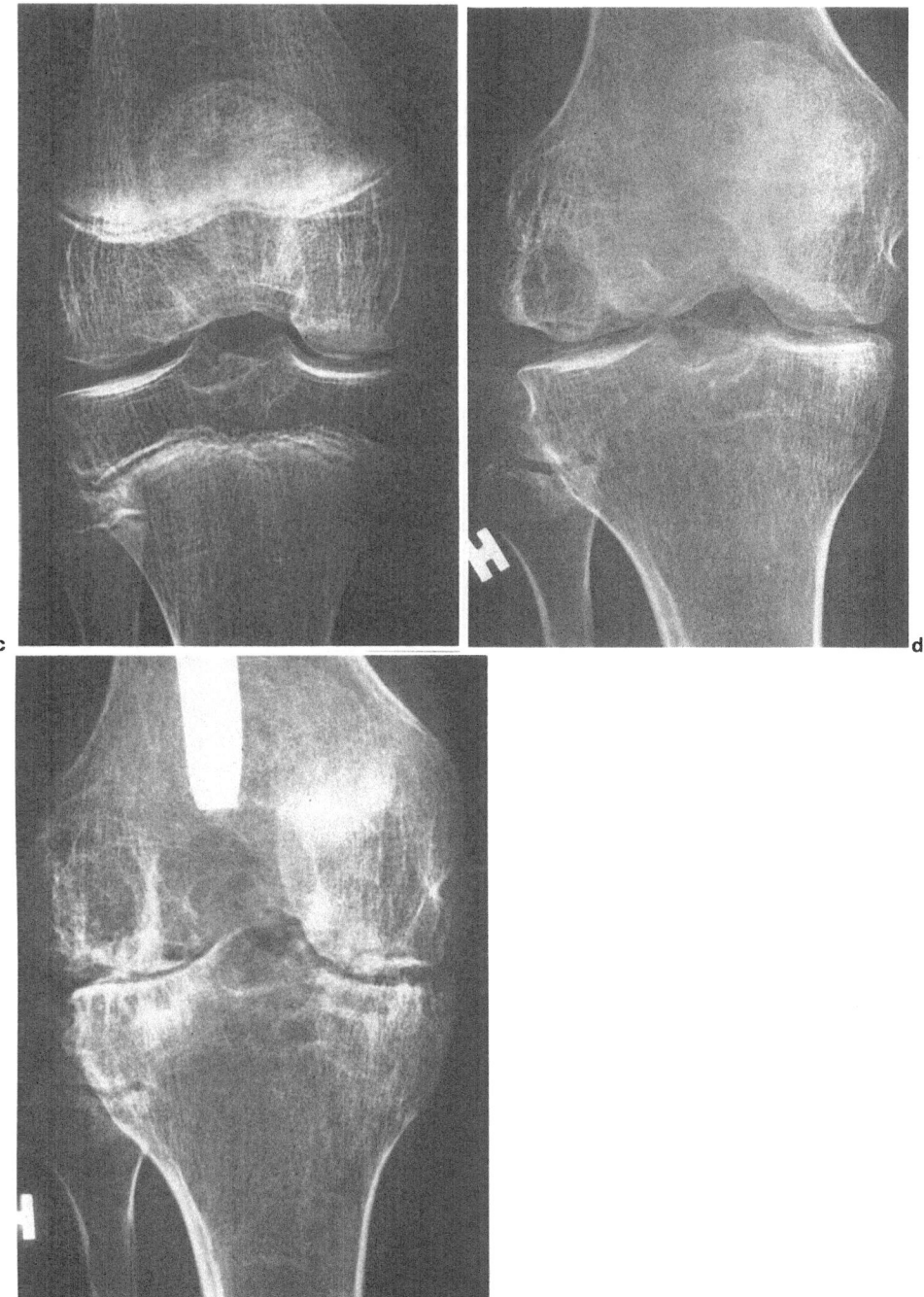

Fig. 3.12a–e. Progression of arthropathy at a knee. A series of views in the same patient at different ages. **a** 7 years old; **b** 12 years old; **c** 17 years old; **d** 24 years old; **e** 30 years old.

Changes Typical for Specific Joints

The radiologic appearance of the arthropathy is basically the same in all joints, but different parts of the mosaic comprising the hemophiliac arthropathy may dominate, giving patterns that are peculiar to each joint.

Shoulder. In the early stages, a tense hemarthrosis may lead to pronounced distention, giving the radiologic appearance of subluxation. Degenerative changes include loss of the cartilaginous joint surface and subchondral cyst formation. As it is a non-weight-bearing joint, subchondral bone collapse is not a common finding. Osteophyte formation, especially at the inferior margin of the glenoid and humeral head, may be pronounced, which is unusual in other joints (Fig. 3.13).

Growth disturbances of the humeral head have often been noticed. These disturbances may include enlargement as in other joints, but an end stage with a small atrophic humeral head is more common (Fonio and Buhler 1952). This small humeral head may be combined with a varus deformity (Fig. 3.14). The reason for these deformities remains unclear, but they are probably due to epiphyseal damage.

An unusual finding that we have noted only at the shoulder is the presence of several large cysts adjacent to both sides of the growth plate (Fig. 3.15). In two cases followed by us they were associated with severe pain.

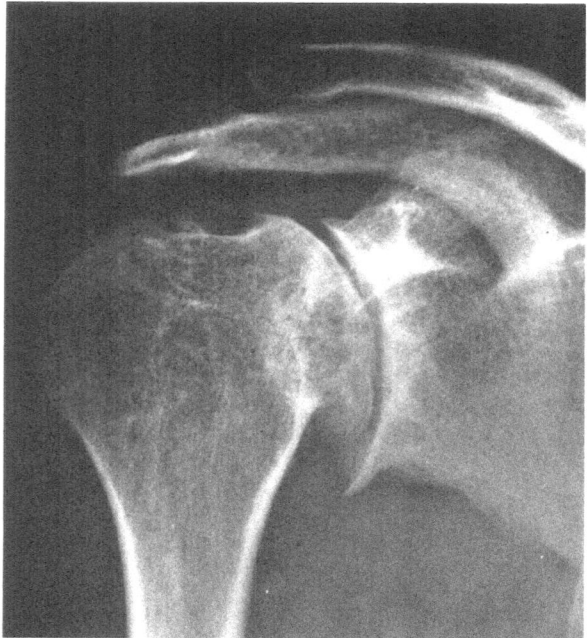

Fig. 3.13. Osteophyte formation and erosions at the shoulder. 31-year-old with severe hemophilia A. In the glenohumeral joint the osteophyte formation may be more pronounced than in other joints. Note the erosion in the cranial part of the humeral head.

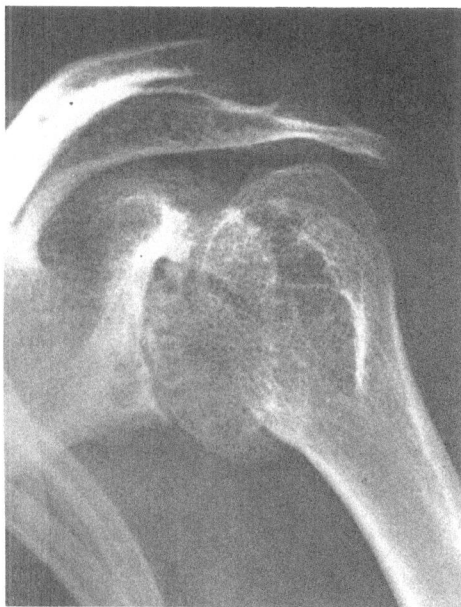

Fig. 3.14. Advanced hemophilic arthropathy of the shoulder. 35-year-old with severe hemophilia A. The humeral head is small, and there is a pronounced varus deformity. The cartilage is destroyed, and there are several small subchondral cysts.

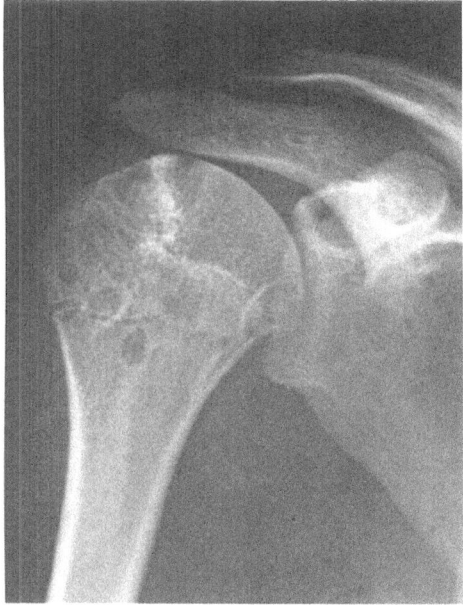

Fig. 3.15. Cyst formation around the growth plate of the shoulder. 18-year-old with severe hemophilia B. In the proximal humerus, cysts adjacent to both sides of the growth plate have been observed with only slight joint destruction.

Elbow. Growth disturbances are common at this joint, with early appearance of ossification centers (Fig. 3.5). The radial head appears early at the affected joint, and, as first described by Shaw (1897), the acceleration may progress to enlargement with incongruity (Fig. 3.16). This may be followed by enlargement of the radial notch of the ulna. In the lateral view this notch may mimic a large irregular cyst with a sclerotic margin, while the AP view will reveal the nature of the lesion (Fig. 3.17).

The distal humerus is enlarged and broadened, and the olecranon fossa is increased in size with its osseous wall often resorbed, producing an olecranon foramen (Fig. 3.18) (Perry 1978). Benz (1980) also has reported on a "radial fossa" of the humerus, adjacent to the olecranon fossa and secondary to radial head enlargement.

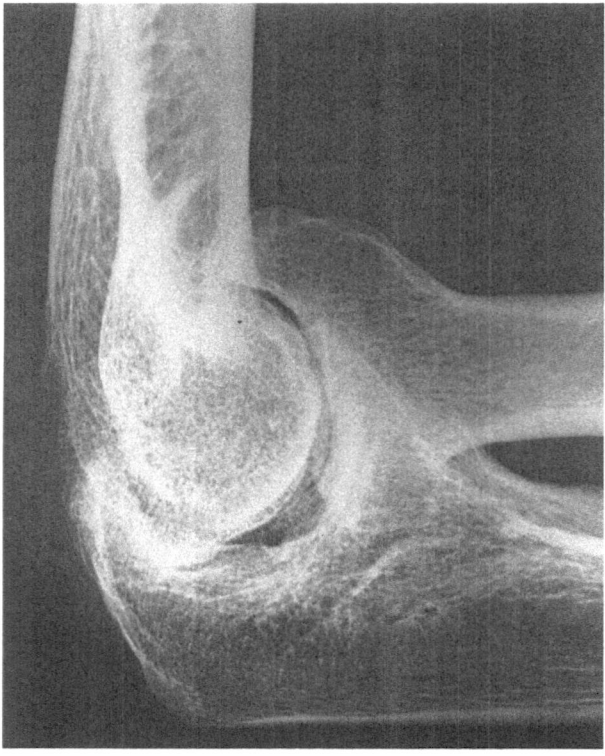

Fig. 3.16. Pronounced enlargement of the radial head. 26-year-old with moderate hemophilia A. The enlargement of the radial head and the proximal ulna may cause an incongruity in the proximal radioulnar joint, with a decreased range of pronation and supination.

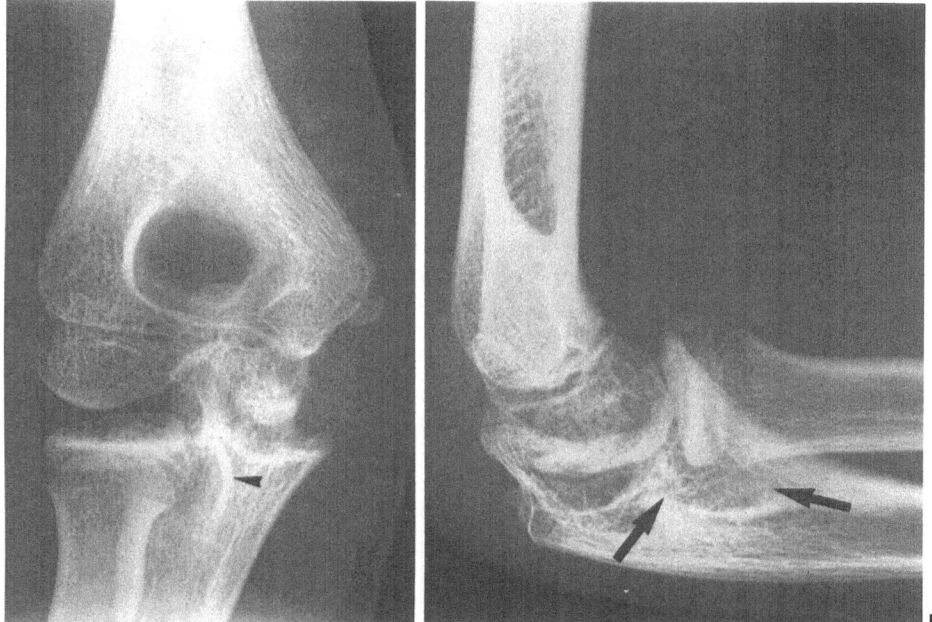

a   b

Fig. 3.17a,b. Enlargement of the radial notch of the ulna. 8-year-old with severe hemophilia A. There is early ossification and accelerated growth of all ossification centers. The enlargement of the radial head has caused a large radial notch of the ulna. In **b** the lateral view, this may appear as a cyst (*arrows*) but in **a** the AP view the nature of the lesion is clearly seen (*arrowhead*).

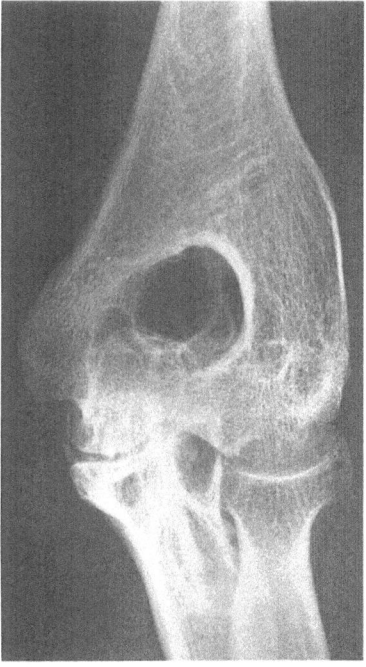

Fig. 3.18. Enlarged olecranon foramen. 22-year-old with severe hemophilia B. The olecranon fossa is enlarged and its wall is resorbed, forming an olecranon foramen.

Subchondral cysts are more common than in other joints, and may become large, especially in the ulna (Fig. 3.19) (Schreiber 1975). Enlargement and pronounced widening of the trochlear notch (Perry 1978) is associated with occasional instability (Fig. 3.20).

As an end result there may be total destruction of the joint, with resorption of the bone ends and luxation (Fig. 3.21), while ankylosis is hardly ever seen.

Wrist. Involvement of the wrist is uncommon. Growth disturbance of the distal end of the ulna causing a luxation of the distal radioulnar joint (Fig. 3.22) has been reported in several patients (Ahlberg 1965), but we have also seen joint space narrowing and subchondral bone destruction (see Fig. 3.32).

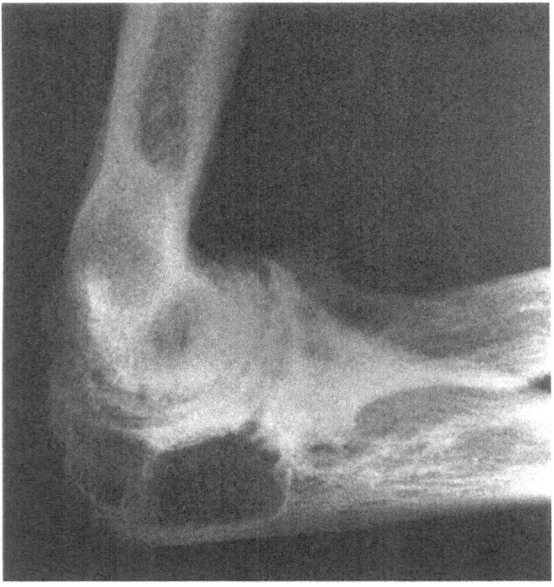

Fig. 3.19. Pronounced subchondral cyst formation in the radius and ulna. 24-year-old with severe hemophilia B. The proximal ulna is enlarged, containing a large cyst system. This is a common site for large cyst formation.

Fig. 3.20a,b. Advanced hemophilic arthropathy in the elbow. 33-year-old with severe hemophilia A. The joint cartilage is totally destroyed, and the bone ends are enlarged and deformed. The trochlear notch is widened, as is the radial notch of the ulna.

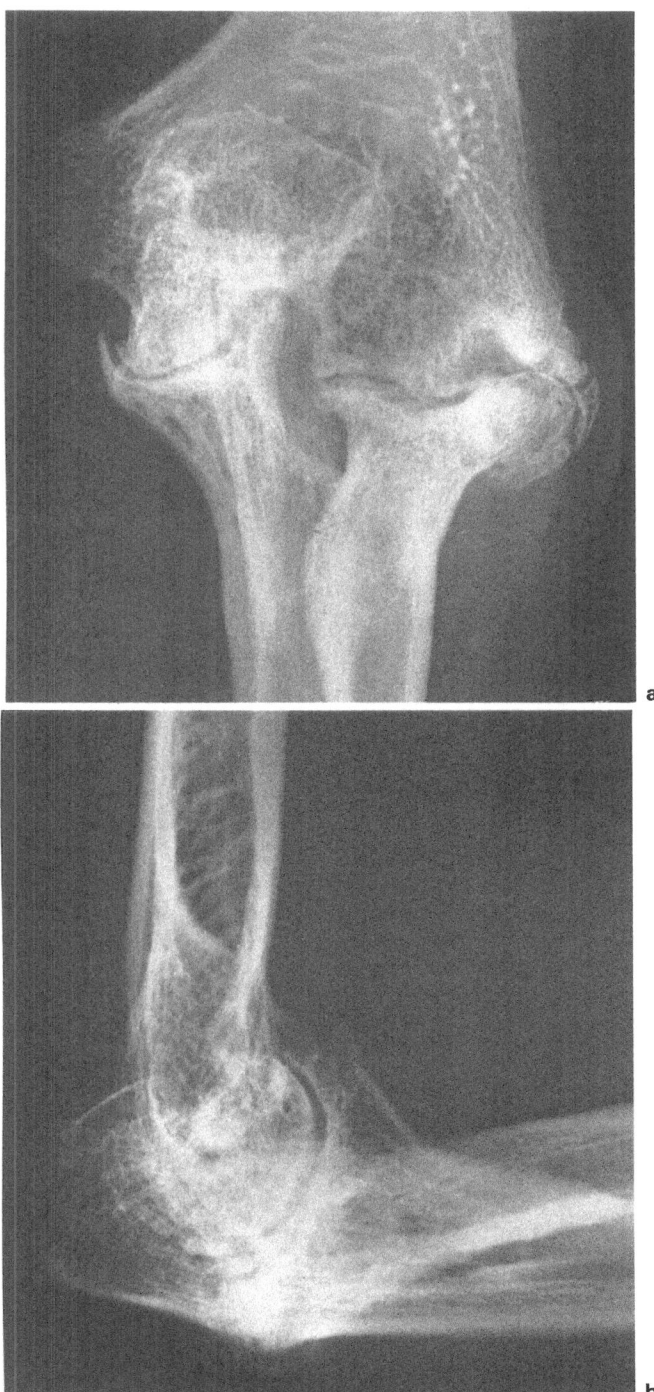

Fig. 3.20.

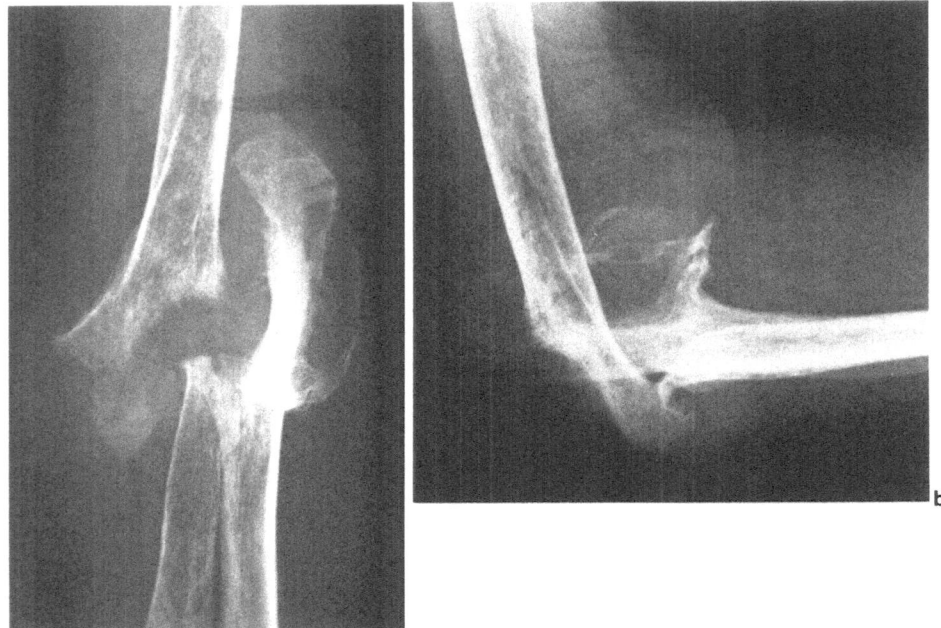

Fig. 3.21a,b. Hemophilic arthropathy of the elbow, end stage. 40-year-old with severe hemophilia A.

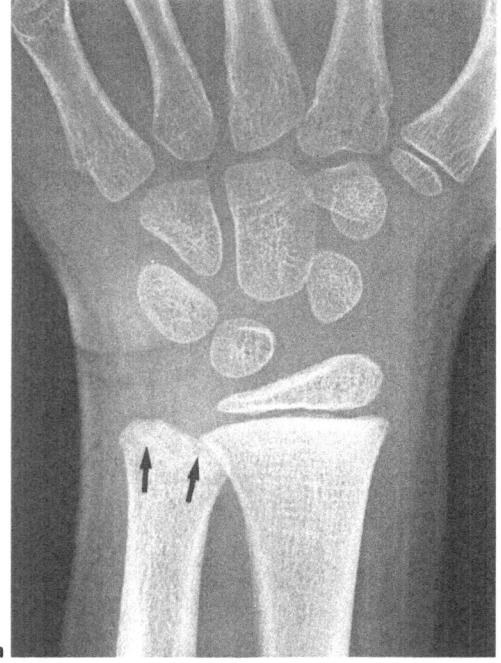

Fig. 3.22.

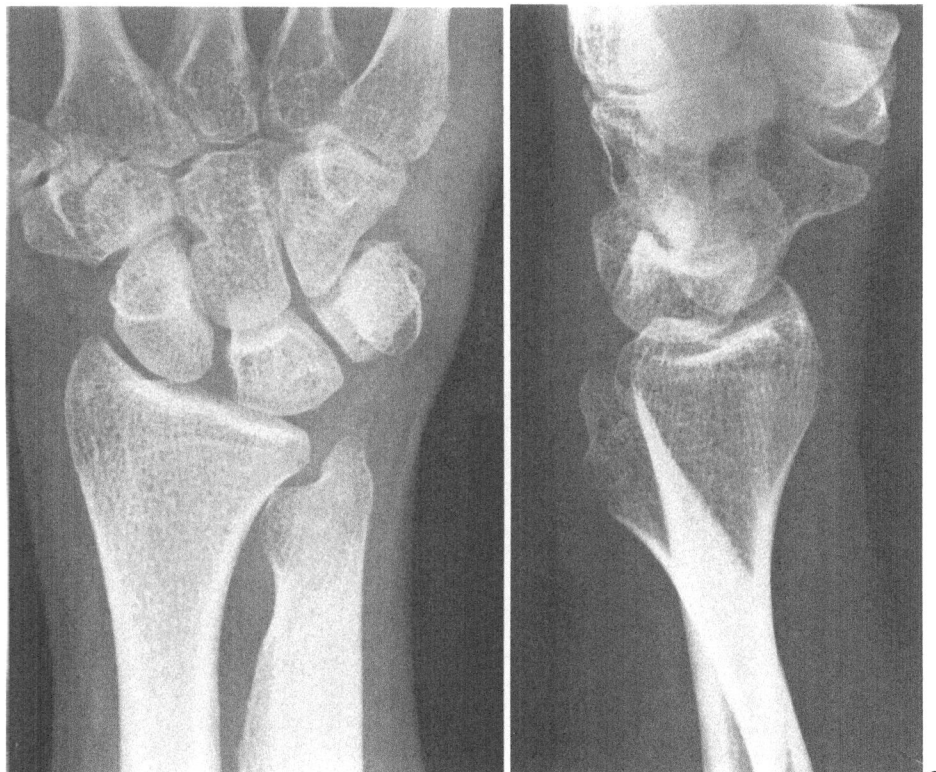

b   c

Fig. 3.22a–c. Development of luxation of the distal radioulnar joint. Severe hemophilia A. **a** At 6 years of age there is an abnormality of the distal ulna. The epiphysis has not ossified, and in the metaphysis there are irregular areas of radiolucency (*arrows*). **b** and **c** At 21 years of age the growth disturbance has resulted in a malformed distal ulna, with luxation of the ulnocarpal and radioulnar joints.

Hip. The final outcome of hemophilic arthropathy of the hip may be dependent on the age of the patient when the hemarthrosis occurred. Thus, according to Winston (1952), hemarthrosis before puberty would result in a radiographic appearance similar to Legg-Calvé-Perthes disease, while hemarthrosis first occurring after puberty would result in a more nonspecific degeneration. However, this age-dependent outcome of the hemarthrosis has not been verified by later authors (Longmaid and Weissman 1982; Wood et al. 1969). The changes, which are similar to avascular necrosis, often involve the whole epiphysis, and the metaphysis is less affected than in classical Legg-Calvé-Perthes disease (Fig. 3.23). The end result may be enlargement of the femoral head (Fig. 3.23c), but resorption and atrophy of the femoral head has also been reported (Fig. 3.24) (Longmaid and Weissman 1982). The current theory is that necrosis of the femoral head is caused by occlusion of epiphyseal vessels secondary to hemarthrosis (Trueta 1963). It has also been suggested that subchondral hemorrhage could be the cause of the epiphyseal necrosis (van Creveld and Kingma 1961), but this is probably very rare (Stoker and Murray 1974).

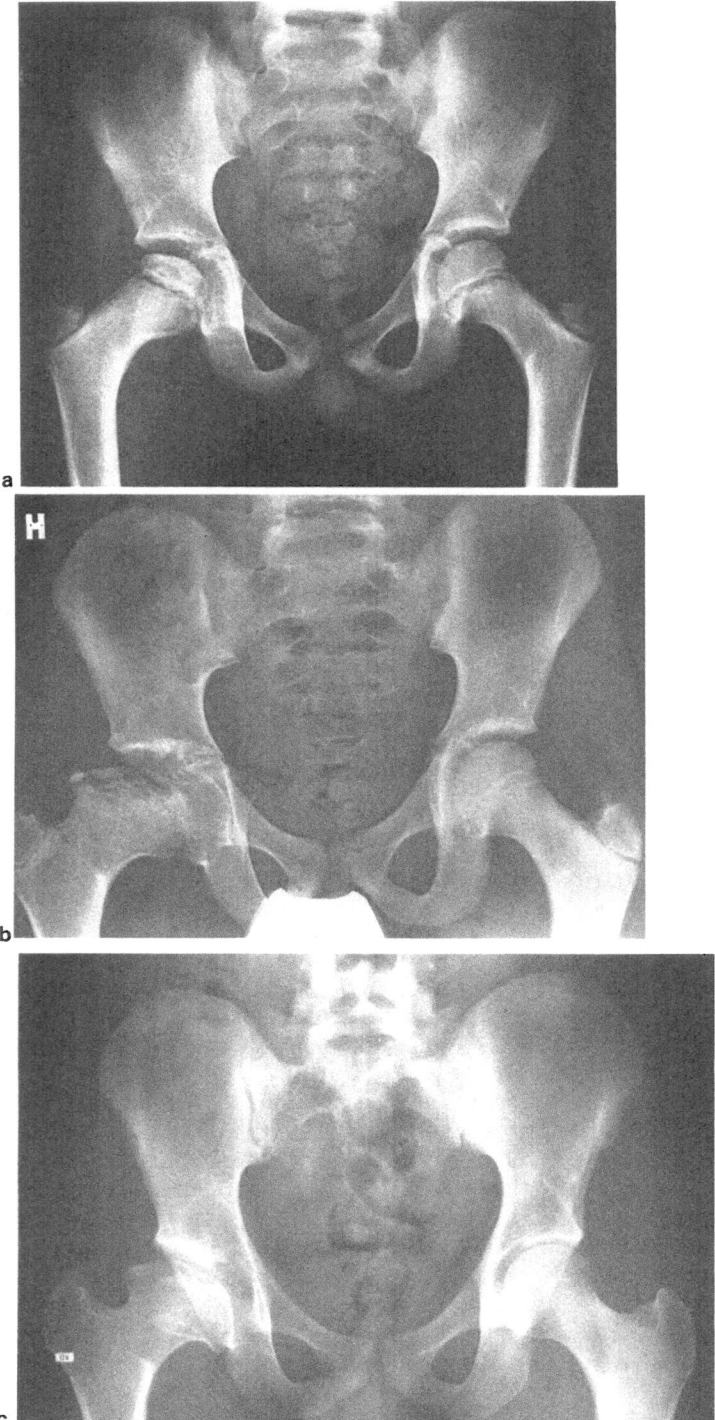

Fig. 3.23.

Fig. 3.23a–c. Legg-Calvé-Perthes-like changes of the right hip. Severe hemophilia A. The same patient at **a** 7, **b** 11, and **c** 19 years of age. The avascular necrosis involves the whole epiphysis. The metaphysis is only slightly irregular but widened.

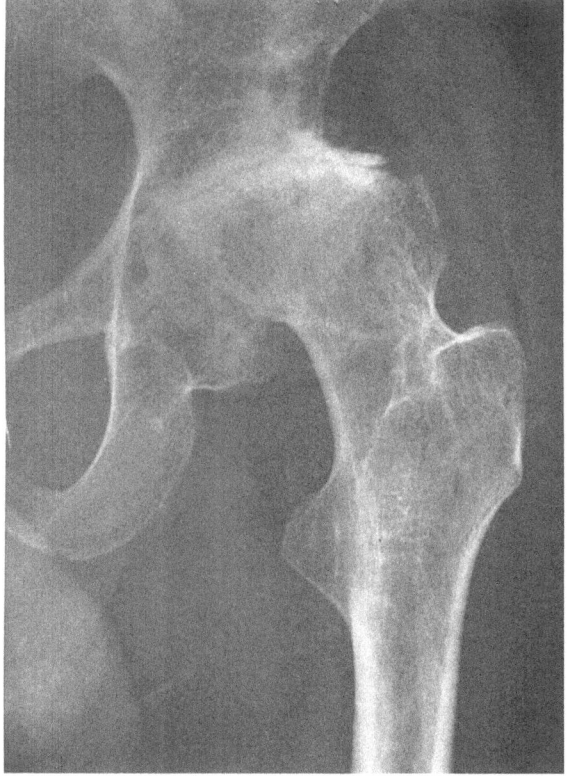

Fig. 3.24. Advanced hemophilic arthropathy of the hip. 36-year-old with severe hemophilia A. In advanced stages there may be atrophy and resorption of the femoral head, with subluxation in the joint.

In advanced cases there may be a central migration of the femoral head into the acetabulum, with thinning of the medial wall of the acetabulum, resulting in a pronounced acetabular protrusion (Schreiber 1975; Teitelbaum 1977).

There are no exact measurements reported on the femoral neck angle, but Teitelbaum (1977) concluded from his material that coxa valga was common. He noted this also in unaffected hips, which is consistent with our experience (Fig. 3.25). These coxa valga might have been caused by disuse of the leg because of affection of the peripheral joints (Stoker and Murray 1974). It is seldom seen today.

Knee. As in the elbow, early manifestations of growth disturbances are common. In small children the ossification center of the patella may appear abnormally early, and its growth may be accelerated (Fig. 3.6c). As an end result, the apex of the patella is flattened, with the characteristic squaring of the lower pole of the patella (Fig. 3.26). Jordan (1958) regarded the squaring of the patella as a consequence of premature cessation of growth, and according to Forrai (1979) the hyperemia associated with chronic inflammation stimulates the fusion between the body of the patella and the ossification center of its lower apex, completing the growth of the bone prematurely. This change was first thought pathognomonic for hemophilia, but later it was shown that the squared patella is more common in juvenile rheumatoid arthritis than in hemophilic arthropathy (Chlosta et al. 1975).

Involvement of the femoropatellar joint is common: diminished joint space, subchondral erosions, cyst formation, and subchondral irregularity parallel the progression of the arthropathy of the femorotibial joint (Leroux et al. 1982) (Figs. 4.4, 4.5).

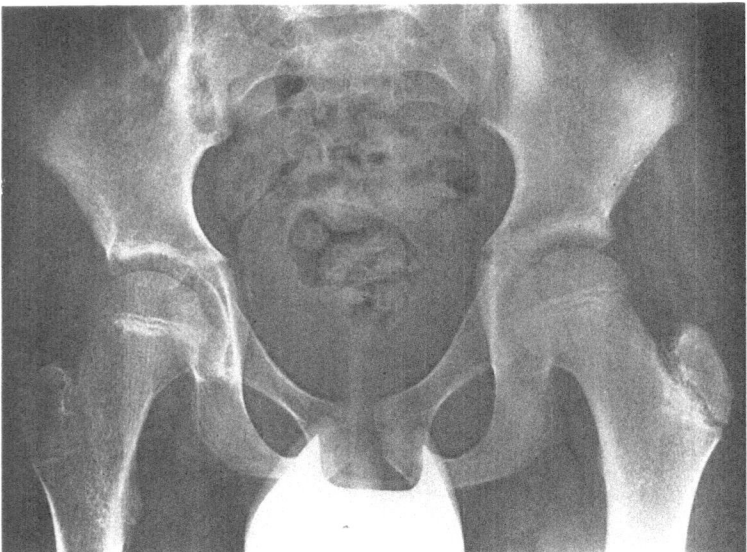

Fig. 3.25. Coxa valga. 12-year-old with severe hemophilia B. Previously, coxa valga was often seen in unaffected hip joints, probably being caused by disuse of the leg because of involvement of the peripheral joints.

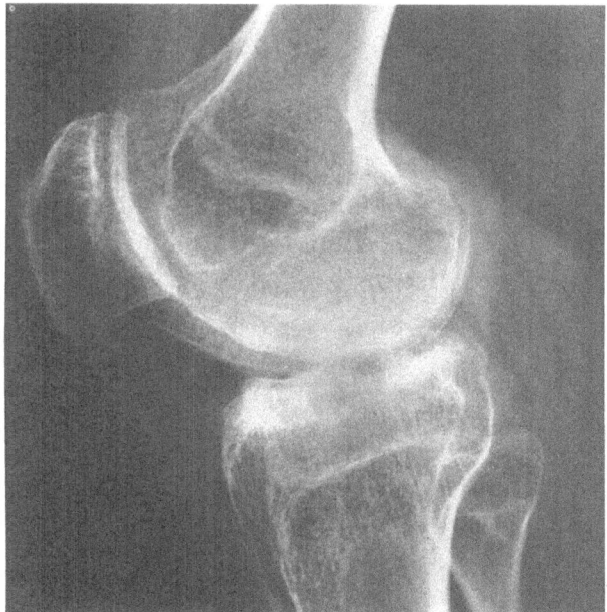

Fig. 3.26. Squaring of the patella. 28-year-old with severe hemophilia B. The patella is enlarged in its anteroposterior diameter, and the lower pole is squared off.

de la Caffiniere et al. (1978) in their study of the patellofemoral syndrome in hemophilic knees also found a high frequency of patellar subluxation and of catching of the patella on a bony "crest" situated at the junction of the trochlea and the condyle of the femur.

Overgrowth of the femoral condyles is common (Figs. 3.6, 3.9). There is also a broadening of the intercondylar notch, which may be caused by overgrowth or by erosions following bleeding at the attachment of the cruciate ligaments (Fig. 3.27). Such broadening was for a long time considered pathognomonic for hemophilic arthropathy (Johnson et al. 1954; Moseley 1963), but the same change may be seen in rheumatoid arthritis, in tuberculosis of the knee joint, and in nonspecific bacterial arthritis (Forrai 1979). Also the groove between the tibial spines may become widened together with the tibial condyles (Fig. 3.27).

In advanced stages, subchondral collapse may cause flattening of the joint surface, and together with severe deformation of the bone ends, posterior subluxation of the tibia results (DePalma 1967) (Figs. 3.9, 3.28). The malalignment may give rise to genu valgum, fixed flexion, and external rotation of the tibia (Fig. 3.28). Ankylosis may also be the end result of hemophilic arthropathy of the knee (Fig. 3.11).

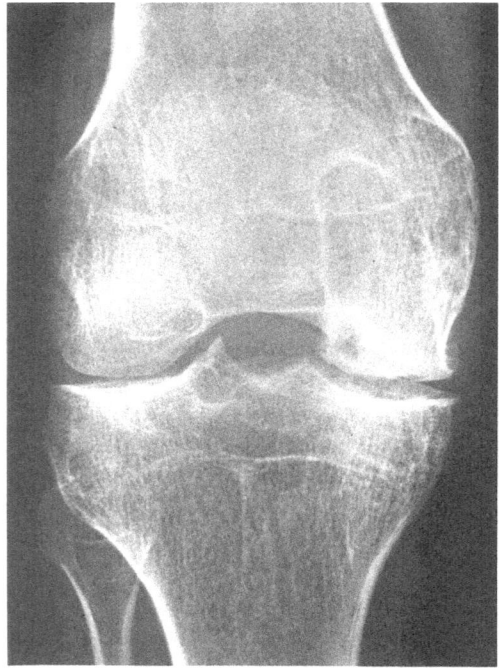

Fig. 3.27. Widening of the femoral intercondylar notch and the groove between the tibial spines. 21-year-old with severe hemophilia A.

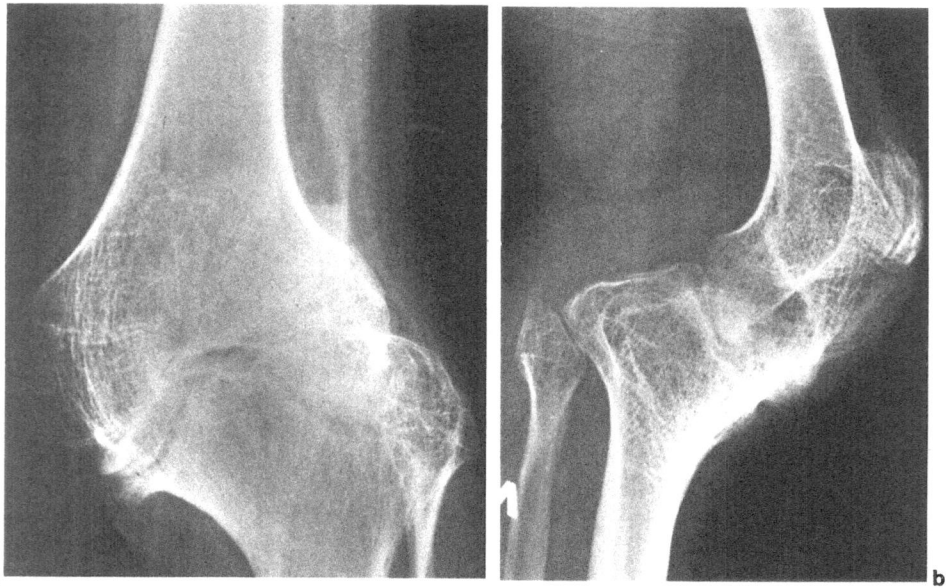

Fig. 3.28a,b. Advanced hemophilic arthropathy of the knee. 33-year-old with severe hemophilia A. There is severe deformation and malalignment of the bone ends, with angulation and posterior subluxation of the tibia. The joint is severely destroyed.

Ankle. Frequently the typical changes are seen at a young age. A common finding in the distal epiphysis of the tibia is narrowing of the lateral part of the epiphysis, with widening medially (Fig. 3.29). This may to some degree be compensated for by deformation of the talar trochlea, which is higher in its lateral than in its medial part (Forrai 1979) (Fig. 3.29). However, these deformations, together with flattening of the joint surface of the talus, may cause valgus deformity of the foot. Total collapse of the body of the talus has been described (Ahlberg 1965; Crock and Boni 1960) (Fig. 3.30). Also ankylosis of the ankle joint has been reported by several authors (Ahlberg 1965; DePalma and Cotler 1956; Fonio and Bühler 1952; Jordan 1958) (Fig. 3.31).

Hands and Feet. Hemophilic arthropathy of the joints in the hands and feet has been regarded as unusual (Heim et al. 1982; Lewis and Sampson 1972), which is in accordance with our experience.

However, in their thorough study of hemophilic arthropathy in the joints of the hands and feet, Pavlov et al. (1979) found frequent involvement of the small joints of the hands and/or feet. The predominating sites were the metacarpophalangeal joints as well as the posterior subtalar joints in the foot. Joint space narrowing, flattening of the subchondral joint surface, and subchondral bone irregularity were the changes most frequently found (Fig. 3.32). We have also found subchondral cyst formation (Fig. 3.33). In the foot, widening of the sinus tarsi, similar to the widening of the intracondylar notch of the femur, has been reported (Zimbler et al. 1976) and ankylosis in the tarsometatarsal joints has been noted (Fig. 3.34). In advanced changes of the ankle and foot there may be a deformity consisting of plantar flexion of the ankle, inversion of the subtalar joints, and adduction of the forefoot (Zimbler et al. 1976) (Fig. 3.35). Advanced changes of the subtalar and talonavicular joints may occur (Fig. 3.30).

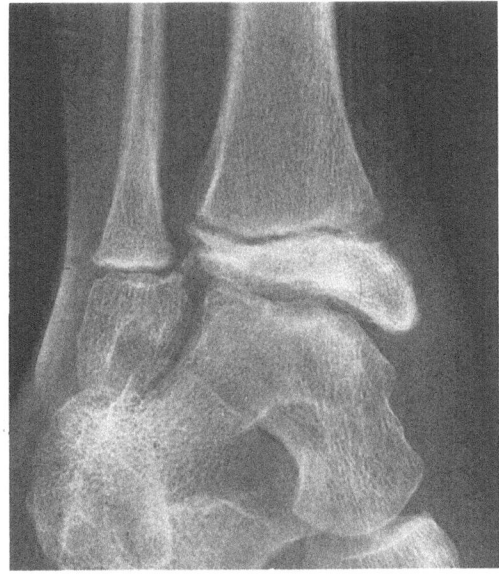

Fig. 3.29. Growth disturbance of the distal epiphysis of the tibia. 8-year-old with severe hemophilia A. The lateral part of the epiphysis is narrowed, while it is widened medially. This appearance is not due to the projection, but is caused by a real growth disturbance. Note also the enlarged fibular epiphysis.

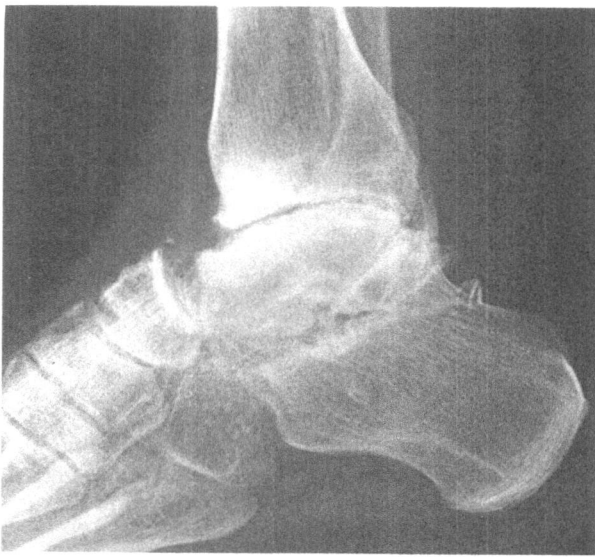

Fig. 3.30. Collapse of the body of the talus. 35-year-old with severe hemophilia A. The talus is irregularly sclerotic, and partially collapsed. Note the advanced arthropathy in the tibiotalar and subtalar joints. The appearance of the talar collapse is to some degree similar to a Charcot joint.

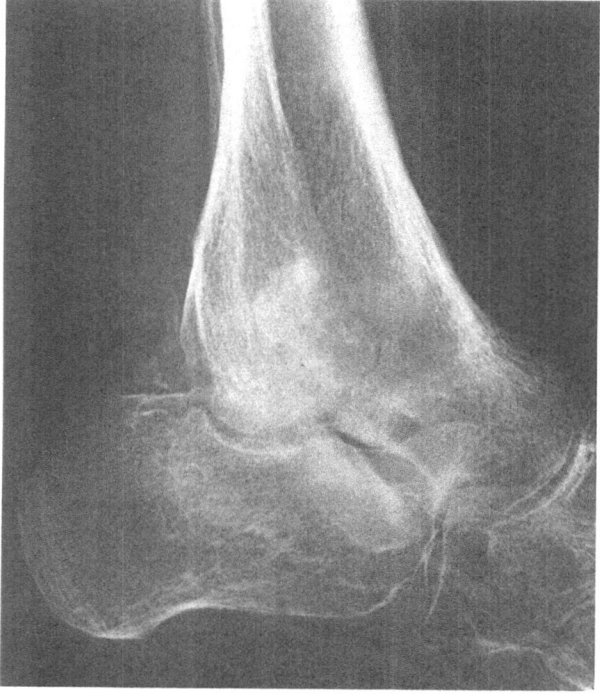

Fig. 3.31. Spontaneous ankylosis of the ankle. 32-year-old with severe hemophilia A. The subtalar joints are preserved.

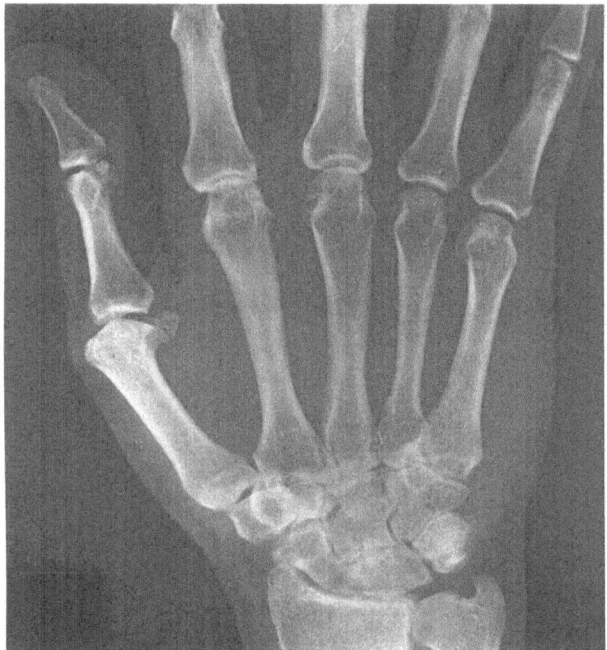

Fig. 3.32. Hemophilic arthropathy of the hand. 25-year-old with severe hemophilia A. There are changes in the wrist, the carpal joints, and the second metacarpophalangeal joint.

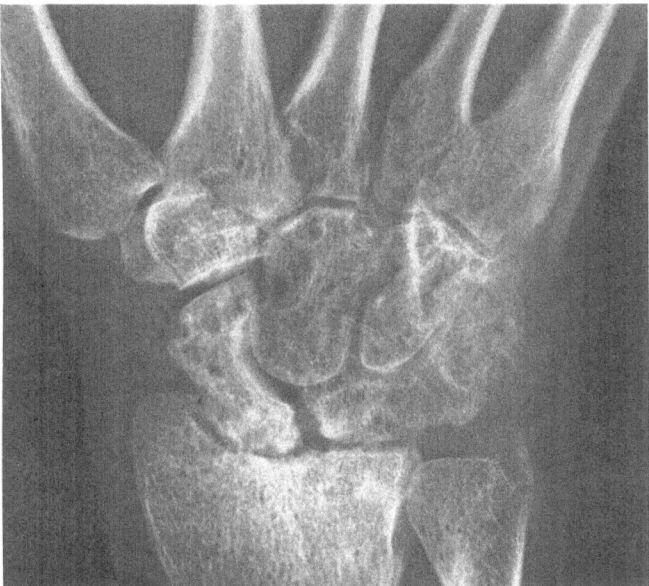

Fig. 3.33. Hemophilic arthropathy of the hand. 30-year-old with severe hemophilia A. Cyst formation in the carpal bones is pronounced.

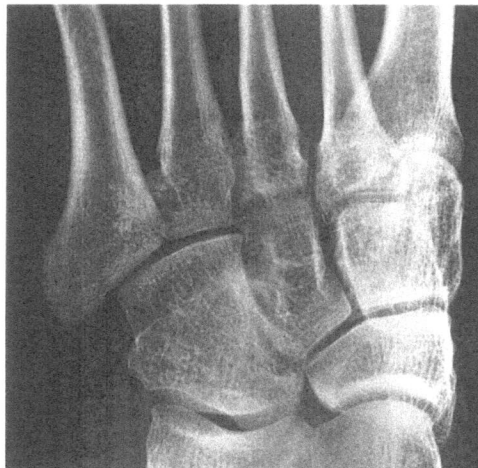

Fig. 3.34. Ankylosis of a tarsometatarsal joint. 20-year-old with severe hemophilia A. This is an unusual site for ankylosis.

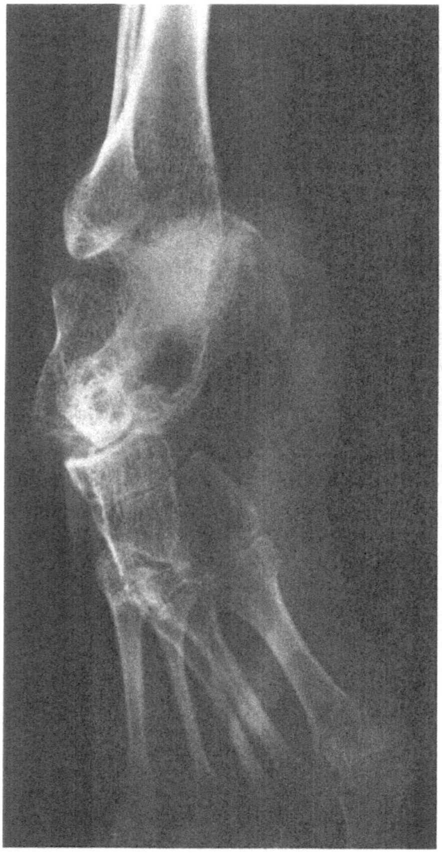

Fig. 3.35a,b. Advanced hemophilic arthropathy of the foot. 22-year-old with severe hemophilia A. There is pronounced plantar flexion, inversion of the subtalar joints, and adduction of the forefoot.

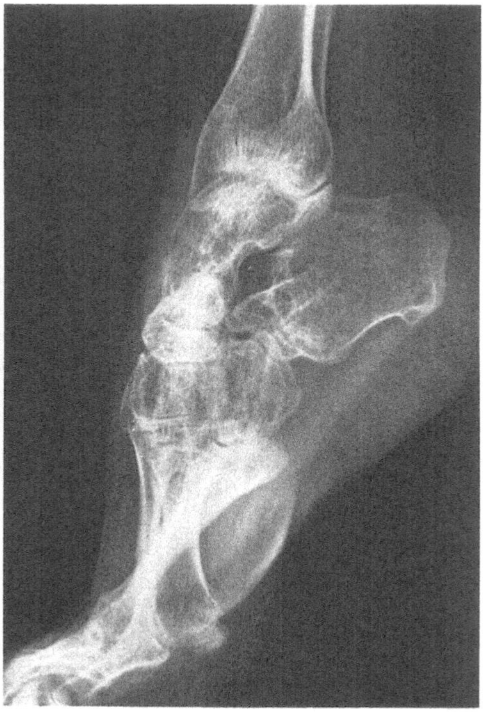

Other Diagnostic Modalities

Arthrography is of limited value in the radiologic evaluation of hemophilic arthropathy. In early stages, the arthrography may be totally normal, and Salerno et al. (1972) found only infrequently synovial irregularity in the examination of nine knees in seven hemophilic children. Compartmentalization of the knee joint has been described by Schreiber (1975).

Computed tomography and *ultrasonography* has been used very rarely for examination of hemophilic arthropathy, but may be of value to differentiate between soft tissue hemorrhage with periarticular soft tissue swelling and hemarthrosis (Fig. 3.36). They may also be used to differentiate between effusion into the joint and synovial thickening.

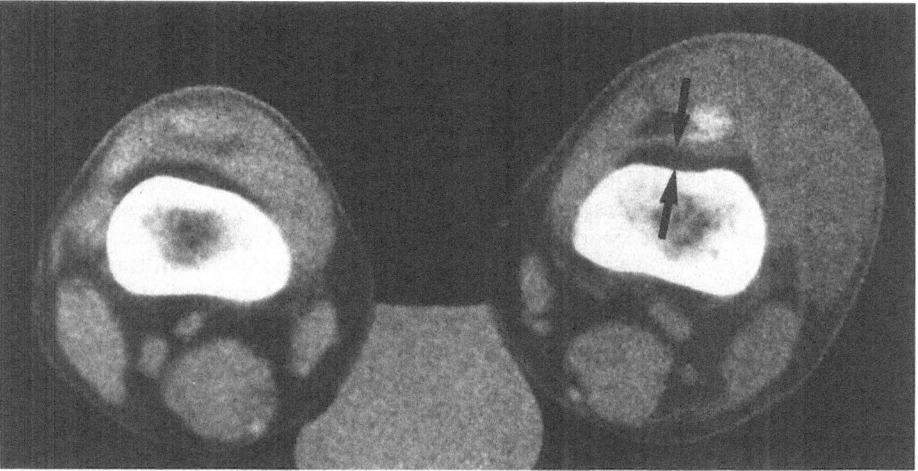

Fig. 3.36. Periarticular soft tissue bleeding, CT examination. 11-year-old with severe hemophilia A. The bleeding into the muscle tissue is obvious and the normal joint space between the patella and the femur is well defined (*arrows*).

The role of *scintimetry* in the assessment of hemophilic arthropathy is small. Although there were publications describing the bone scan appearance of hemophilic arthropathy (Forbes et al. 1972; Cambouroglou et al. 1976; Licata et al. 1977) shortly after bone scanning in benign disease was made possible in the mid 1970s, there has been very little written on the subject since then. In some centers this modality has been used to assess the effect of synoviorthesis with radioactive substances (Fernandez-Pallazi and de Bosch 1983). However, most major institutions have found the role of nuclear medicine in the evaluation of hemophilic arthropathy to be negligible.

At the present time nothing has been reported on the use of *magnetic resonance imaging* in the examination of hemophilic arthropathy. However, as this is being written, and with every passing week, additions are made to the MRI experience. In the future, MRI will probably provide additional information on both the structural and the biochemical changes occurring in hemophilic arthropathy.

Classification of Hemophilic Arthropathy

From the above description of hemophilic arthropathy it is obvious that the joint lesions are manifold, and that the degree of joint destruction is unpredictable even in patients with the same severity of factor deficiency. From a scientific point of view as well as in daily routine work it is necessary to be able to classify the degree of joint destruction in order to study the natural course of the arthropathy and to evaluate the effect of different therapeutic regimes.

Previous Classifications

As mentioned earlier in this chapter, in his thorough description of hemophilic arthropathy König (1892) distinguished between hemarthrosis, panarthritis, and a regressive stage, and Key (1932) simplified this classification to only two stages: acute hemarthrosis and chronic arthritis. DePalma and Cotler (1956) based a classification on a combination of clinical and radiographic findings, and Jordan (1958) designed a very similar classification based mainly on the radiographic changes. These authors proposed four classes of hemophilic joint destruction, the first grade being the earliest and slightest, and the fourth grade, a totally destroyed joint with ankylosis or marked loss of mobility, pronounced deformity, and severe radiologic changes. Ahlberg (1965) based his classification on the grades 2–4 in the DePalma and Cotler system. In 1977 Arnold and Hilgartner designed a five-grade scale based on both radiologic changes and clinical examination in which they claimed good correlation between the radiologic stage and the clinical state.

In 1969 Wood et al. proposed a classification exclusively based on radiographic changes and designed as a score system. But this system included several changes that are seen only in the acute stages of a hemarthrosis, and thus was not suitable for expressing the chronic progression of hemophilic arthropathy.

Modern prophylactic and therapeutic methods require techniques for measuring the severity of joint destruction that are not only objective but also sensitive. Even small changes between two consecutive examinations of a given patient may be important (Ahlberg and Pettersson 1981). Thus a new detailed clinical and radiologic classification of the hemophilic joint, more suited to modern needs, was recommended by the Orthopedic Advisory Committee of the World Federation of Hemophilia after the latter's 1981 meeting; this classification is based on a thorough clinical assessment and on a sensitive radiologic classification previously proposed by Pettersson et al. 1980).

The Classification Recommended by the Orthopedic Advisory Committee of the World Federation of Hemophilia

Clinical Evaluation

The clinical evaluation includes patient data, joint evaluation, and physical examination as detailed below:

I.   *Patient Data*
   1.   Age
   2.   Factor deficiency
        (VIII, IX, etc.)
   3.   Factor level
   4.   Inhibitor?
        (Yes or No)
   5.   Mode of treatment
        O   = No, or minimal transfusion therapy
        E   = Episodic transfusion for most or all bleeding episodes
        M   = Maintenance or prophylactic therapy
        (H)   = Added after E or M indicates that the patient is on a home or
                self-transfusion program

Example: 16:VIII: <1:No:E(H)
A 16-year-old patient, factor VIII deficient, with a level of less than 1%. He does
not have an inhibitor and treats at home on an episodic basis.

II.   *Joint Evaluation* (of the nonbleeding joint)
   1.   Pain
        0–3
   2.   Bleeding
        0–3
   3.   Physical examination
        0–12
   4.   Radiologic evaluation
        0–13

   If the limb described requires an aid to ambulation, the following letters
   should be added at the end of the evaluation:

        B   = Brace or orthosis
        C   = Cane
        CR   = Crutches
        WC = Wheelchair

PAIN

   0: No pain
       No functional deficit
       No analgesic use (except with acute hemarthrosis)
   1: Mild pain
       Does not interfere with occupation nor with activities of daily living
       (ADL)
       May require occasional non-narcotic analgesic
   2: Moderate pain
       Partial or occasional interference with occupation or ADL
       Use of non-narcotic medications
       May require occasional narcotics

3: Severe pain
   Interferes with occupation or ADL
   Requires frequent use of non-narcotic and narcotic medications

BLEEDING

This is measured by the number of minor and major hemarthroses *per year*.

0   = None
1   = No major, 1–3 minor
2   = 1–2 major or 4–6 minor
3   = 3 or more major or 7 or more minor

Guidelines:

Minor	*Major*
Mild pain	Pain
Minimal swelling	Effusion
Minimal restriction of motion	Limitation of motion
Resolves within 24 h of treatment	Failure to respond within 24 h

PHYSICAL EXAMINATION

This is based on an additive score of 0–12 with 0 being a normal joint and 12 being most affected. An (S) is added after the number if a chronic synovitis is clinically diagnosed.

Swelling	0 or 2 + (S)
Muscle atrophy	0–1
Axial deformity	0–2
Crepitus on motion	0–1
Range of motion	0–2
Flexion contracture	0 or 2
Instability	0–2

Guidelines:

Swelling:

0   = None
2   = Present
(S) = Added after score if chronic synovitis is present

Muscle atrophy:

0   = None or minimal (< 1 cm)
1   = Present

Axial deformity (measured only at knee or ankle):

Knee:

0   = Normal = 0–7° valgus
1   =   8–15° valgus or 0–5° varus
2   =   > 15° valgus or > 5° varus

Ankle:

0   = No deformity

1   = Up to 10° valgus or up to 5° varus

2   = > 10° valgus or > 5° varus

Crepitus on motion:

0   = None

1   = Present

Range of motion:

0   = Loss of 10% of total full range of motion (FROM)

1   = Loss of 10–33⅓% of total FROM

2   = Loss of > 33⅓% of total FROM

Flexion contracture:

Measured only at hip, knee, or ankle

0   = < 15° FFC (fixed flexion contracture)

2   = 15° or greater FFC at hip or knee or equinus at ankle

Instability:

0   = None

1   = Noted on examination but neither interferes with function nor requires bracing

2   = Instability that creates a functional deficit or requires bracing

Radiologic Evaluation

The radiologic classification is that designed by Pettersson et al. (1980), which was based on a retrospective investigation of the radiographs of 54 patients with hemophilia A or B who were admitted to the International Hemophilia Treatment and Training Center in Malmö, Sweden. When first seen at the Center, their ages ranged from 9 months to 25 years. All patients had had radiologic examination of the large joints (shoulders, elbows, wrists, hips, knees, and ankles), and 24 of them had follow-up radiologic examination 2–18 years later, before the institution of any specific therapeutic or prophylactic treatment. In all, about 1000 radiographs were reviewed.

First, any changes attributed to hemophilic arthropathy were assessed: intra-articular effusion, periarticular soft tissue thickening, periarticular soft tissue calcification, synovial thickening and increased density, enlargement of the ossified parts of the epiphyses, periarticular osteoporosis, narrowed joint space, irregularity of subchondral surfaces, subchondral sclerosis, subchondral cysts, incongruity of articular surfaces, erosions of joint margins, Harris' lines, angulation or/and displacement of articulating bones, and ankylosis. Of these changes, those which could be measured radiologically and which were not attributed to any recent occurrence of bleeding were selected for further study.

Joint swelling might be caused by recent bleeding and thus was omitted. Assessment of soft tissue thickening, calcification, synovial thickening, and increased density proved very dependent on the technique used at the examination, making comparison from one examination to another unreliable. Therefore these changes,

Table 3.2. Radiologic evaluation recommended by the Orthopedic Advisory Committee of the World Federation of Hemophilia

Type of change	Finding	Score (points)
Osteoporosis	Absent	0
	Present	1
Enlarged epiphysis	Absent	0
	Present	1
Irregular subchondral surface	Absent	0
	Partly involved	1
	Totally involved	2
Narrowing of joint space	Absent	0
	Joint space > 1 mm	1
	Joint space ≤ 1 mm	2
Subchondral cyst formation	Absent	0
	1 cyst	1
	> 1 cyst	2
Erosions of joint margins	Absent	0
	Present	1
Gross incongruence of articulating bone ends	Absent	0
	Slight	1
	Pronounced	2
Joint deformity (angulation and/or displacement between articulating bones)	Absent	0
	Slight	1
	Pronounced	2
Possible joint score: 0–13 points		

all used in the classification of Wood et al. (1969), were also omitted. Subchondral sclerosis appeared to be a component of subchondral irregularity or cyst formation, as already described by DePalma (1967), and was not taken into account. As has been described earlier, Harris' lines are totally nonspecific, and thus were not included. The remaining changes were recorded in a chronologic order of occurrence, and each change was allotted 0–2 points according to its existence and severity (Table 3.2). The sum of points allotted to a given joint at each examination was said to be the *joint score*. The sum of the joint scores obtained from the 12 great joints constituted the *patient score*. It has subsequently appeared that as the shoulder joints and the hips are seldom affected, a patient score *based on assessment of elbows, knees, and ankles* is equally reliable for scientific purposes or for assessment of the effect of therapeutic regimens, and thus should be preferred.

Examples of Use of the Radiologic Classification

1. *The Natural Course of Hemophilic Arthropathy.* Using the radiologic classification it is possible to express the natural course of hemophilic arthropathy in single joints, single patients, or patient groups. In a retrospective investigation we reviewed the 54 patients defined above, with severe and moderate hemophilia A or B, who had had repeated radiographic examination of all large joints (shoulder, elbow, hip, knee, ankle) during the 1950s and 60s, before institution of any specific treatment. Using the present radiologic classification, the joint score was assessed in all patients. In 24 of the patients it was also possible to follow the joint and patient scores for periods varying between 2 and 18 years. Figure 3.37 shows the

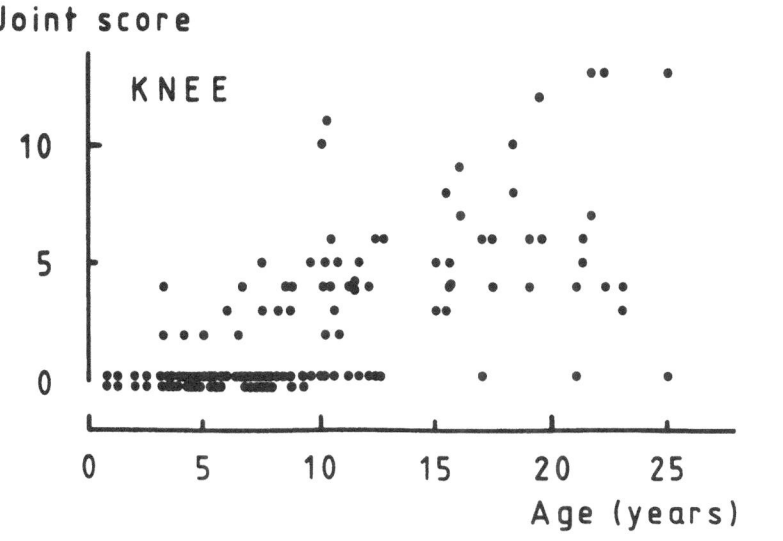

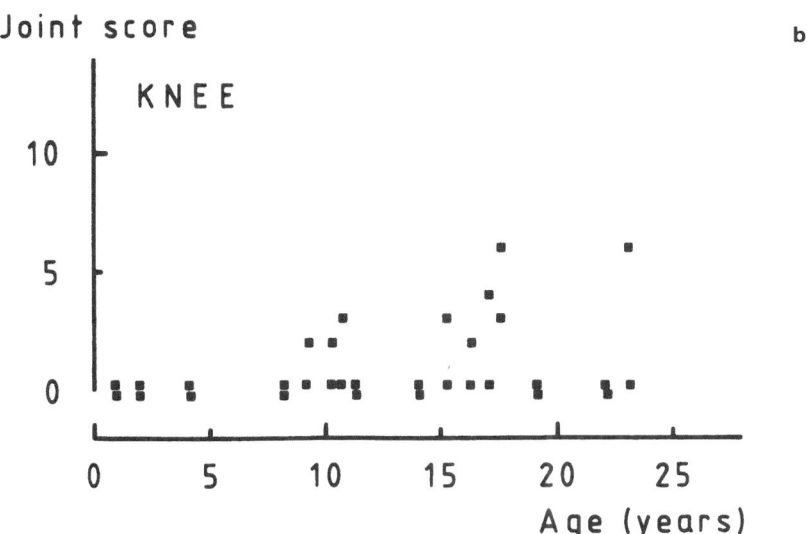

Fig. 3.37. Joint score of the knees according to age, obtained in 54 patients with **a** severe and **b** moderate hemophilia, examined before the institution of any specific treatment. (From Pettersson et al. 1980, with permission.)

joint score obtained in the knees. It is obvious that the severity of the arthropathy increased with age, and that the changes occurred later and were less pronounced in moderate than in severe hemophilia. No changes were seen below the age of 3 years. Unaffected joints were noted in all ages. Figure 3.38 gives the patient score according to age at all examinations reviewed, and Fig. 3.39 the course of the

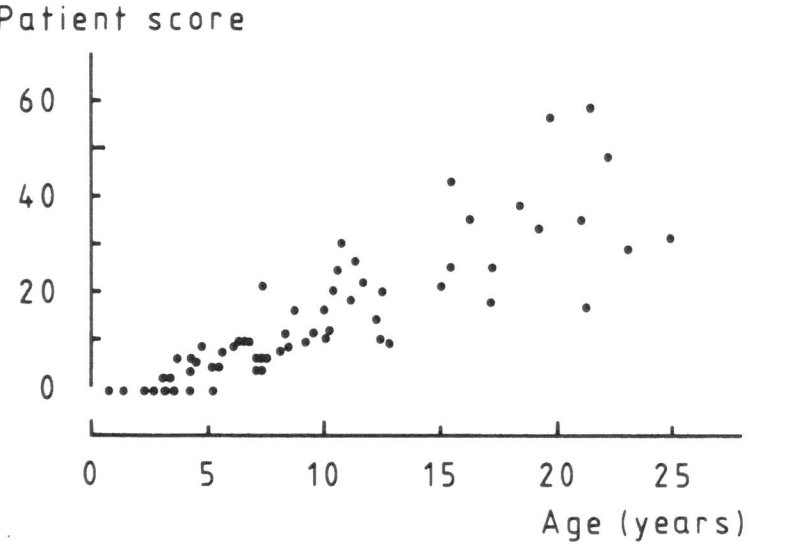

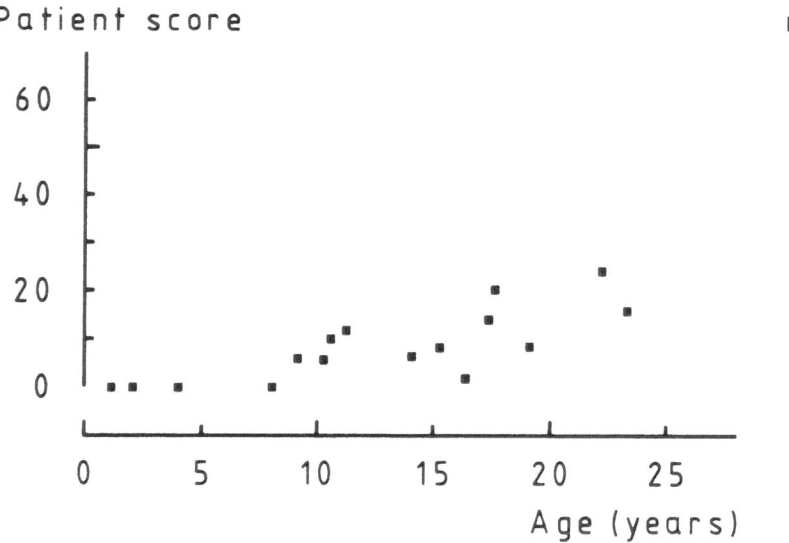

Fig. 3.38. Patient score according to age obtained in 54 patient patients with **a** severe and **b** moderate hemophilia, examined before the institution of any specific treatment. (From Pettersson et al. 1980, with permission.)

patient score in those followed for 2–18 years. In severe hemophilia no patient had a score above zero before the age of 3 years, whereas no child aged 6 or more was free from radiologic changes. Children with moderate hemophilia were affected later and less severely. In no patient except those with a score of zero were the

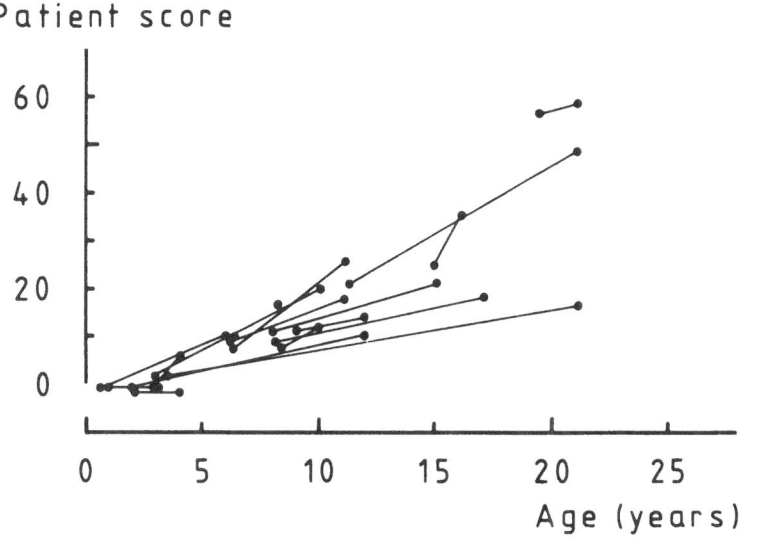

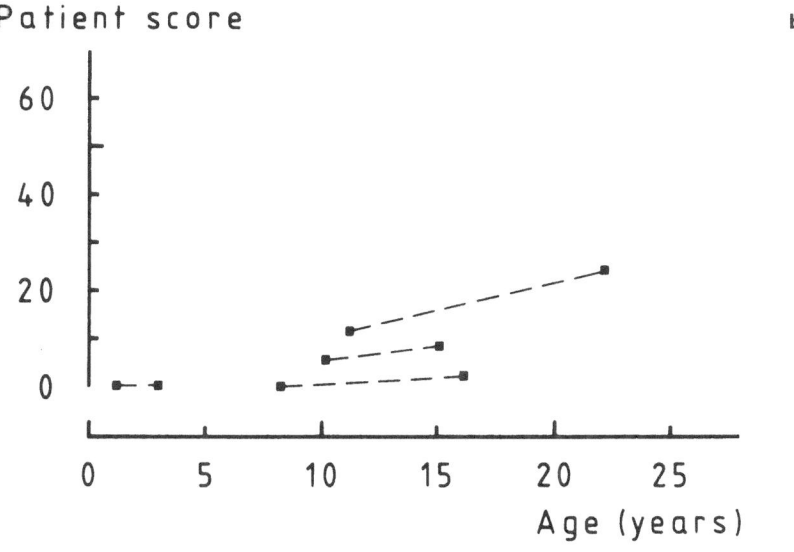

Fig. 3.39. The natural course of the patient score in patients with **a** severe and **b** moderate hemophilia, followed for 2–18 years before the institution of any specific treatment. (From Pettersson et al. 1980, with permission.)

changes stationary. The increase with time was more rapid in severe than in moderate hemophilia. In Fig. 3.40 the patients have been divided into age groups with 5-year intervals. The increase in patients' scores with age is fairly constant, although the progression may be slightly less pronounced after the age of 20 years.

Mean patient score

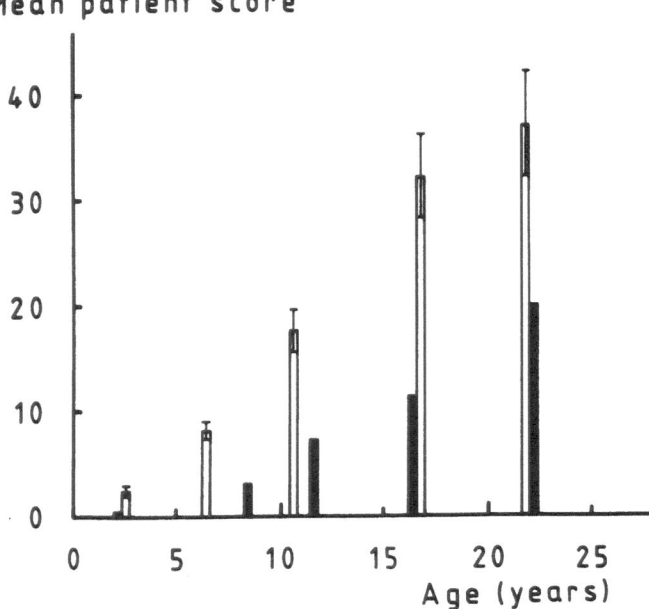

Fig. 3.40. Mean patient score according to age in 54 patients with severe or moderate hemophilia, examined before the institution of any specific treatment. The patients are divided into age groups with 5-year intervals. *Open area* = severe hemophilia; *black area* = moderate hemophilia; *I* = standard error of mean. (From Pettersson et al. 1980, with permission.)

2. *Assessment of the Effect of Modern Treatment and Prophylaxis.* Knowing the natural course in terms of the classification, it is possible to evaluate the effect of prophylaxis (Nilsson et al. 1981; Pettersson et al. 1981) or to assess the effect of therapeutic efforts in selected joints (Ahlberg and Pettersson 1981; Heijnen et al. 1983).

In a recent investigation (Pettersson and Nilsson 1984) 45 patients with severe hemophilia A, on prophylaxis for 1–18 years, were followed with clinical and radiologic examinations. The patients were divided into age groups with 5-year intervals as described above. The mean patient score in each age group was calculated and compared with the values found for the natural course of the disease (Fig. 3.41). It is obvious that the prophylaxis has changed the mean score from that of severe hemophilia during the natural course to that of moderate hemophilia. In the lower age groups the prophylaxis has been instituted at a very low age. We have earlier shown that during prophylaxis very few new joints are involved, the main part of the progression being due to destruction in already affected joints (Pettersson et al. 1982). To be really effective, prophylaxis should start at a very young age, presumably about 2 years.

Mean patient score

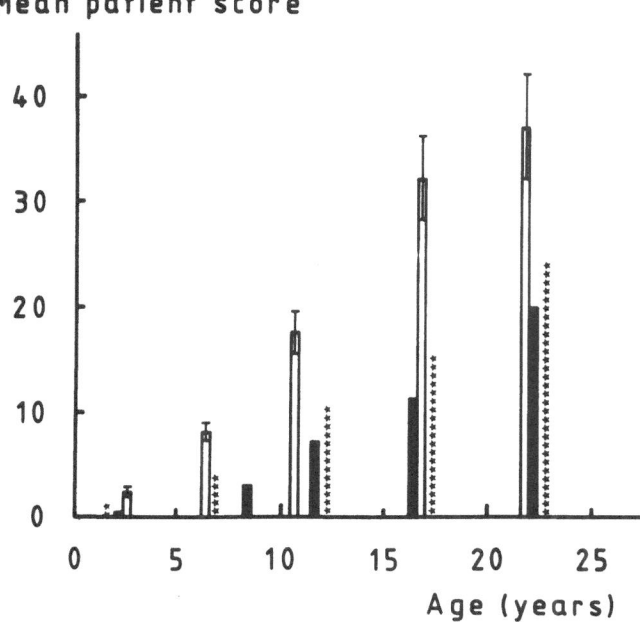

Fig. 3.41. Mean patient score according to age in 45 patients with severe hemophilia A, on prophylaxis for 1–18 years, compared with the mean patient score according to age during the natural course of the disease (compare Fig. 3.40). *Open area* = severe hemophilia, natural course; *black area* = moderate hemophilia, natural course; *starred area* = severe hemophilia, during prophylaxis.

The Relevance of the Radiologic Classification

A radiologic classification suitable for a thorough assessment of hemophilic arthropathy should fulfil the following criteria:

1. It should be objective, with high reproducibility and accuracy.
2. The changes considered should not be caused by an ongoing bleeding, but be relevant for the long-term progression of the arthropathy.
3. The changes should be quantifiable.
4. It should measure the arthropathy in a single joint, a single patient, or a group of joints or patients.
5. It should be based on standard radiographs, easily obtainable at any hemophilic treatment center.

To test the inter- and intraobserver variation of the method, two experienced radiologists classified the ten large joints of 50 patients on two different occasions, at an interval of 6 months. It was found that for the patient score the intraobserver variation was 3 points with a statistical significance of $P<0.05$ and 4 points with $P<0.01$. The interobserver variation was 5 points with a statistical significance of $P<0.05$ and 7 points with $P<0.01$. Heijnen et al. (1983) have shown that the intra- and interobserver variation for individual joints is very small.

The State of the Joint in Terms of the Clinical and Radiologic Evaluation

Using the scoring system presented, both for the clinical evaluation and the radiologic classification, the state of the joint may be expressed in short terms, making it easy to compare from one time to another in the same patient, or to compare patients.

Examples:

1. 1:1:5(S):4 is a joint with mild pain, minimal bleeding, and moderate changes on physical examination. A synovitis is present and the radiologic changes are moderate.

2. 3:3:10:9:B is a joint that is painful and bleeds often. The changes on physical examination and X-ray are severe and the patient uses a brace to walk.

References

Ahlberg Å (1965) Haemophilia in Sweden. VII. Incidence, treatment and prophylaxis of arthropathy and other musculoskeletal manifestations of haemophilia A and B. Acta Orthop Scand (Suppl) 77

Ahlberg Å, Pettersson H (1981) Radiologic examination for follow-up of haemophilic arthropathy. In: Seligsohn U, Rimon A, Horoszowski H (eds) Haemophilia. Castle House, London, pp 175–181

Arnold WD, Hilgartner MW (1977) Hemophilic arthropathy. Current concepts of pathogenesis and management. J Bone Joint Surg [Am] 59: 287–305

Aronstam A, Rainsfad SG, Painter MJ (1979) Patterns of bleeding in adolescents with severe hemophilia A. Br Med J I: 467–472

Benz HJ (1980) The development of epiphyses in hemophiliac arthropathy of the elbow. RÖFO 133: 305–311

Brown IS, Toolis F, Prescott RJ (1982) Haemophilic arthropathy: A ten year radiologic and clinical study. Scott Med J 27: 279–283

Caffey J, Schlesinger ER (1940) Certain effects of hemophilia on the growing skeleton: Some roentgenographic observations on overgrowth and dysgenesis of the epiphyses associated with chronic hemarthrosis. J Pediatr 16: 549–565

Cambouroglou G, Papathanassiou B, Koutoulidis C, Bossinakou I, Mandalaki T (1976) Haemophilic arthropathy surveyed with whole-body gamma-camera scintigraphy. Acta Orthop Scand 47: 607–612

Chlosta EM, Kuhns LR, Holt JF (1975) The "patellar ratio" in hemophilia and juvenile rheumatoid arthritis. Radiology 116: 137–138

Crock HV, Boni V (1960) The management of orthopaedic problems in haemophiliacs. A review of 21 cases. Br J Surg 48: 8–14

de la Caffiniere JY, Allain JP, Laurian Y, Larrieu MJ (1978) Patello-femoral syndrome in hemophiliac knee. Acta Orthop Belg 44: 389–401

DePalma AF (1967) Hemophilic arthropathy. Clin Orthop 52: 145–165

DePalma AF, Cotler JM (1956) Hemophilic arthropathy. Arch Surg 72: 247–250

Duthie RB, Stein H (1977) Ultrastructural changes in microprobe analysis of haemophilic joint tissues. J Bone Joint Surg [Br] 59: 118

Duthie RB, Matthews JM, Rizza CR, Steel WM (1972) The management of musculo-skeletal problems in the haemophilias. Blackwell, Oxford

Fernandez-Pallazi F, de Bosch NB (1983) Radioactive synoviorthesis in hemophilic hemarthrosis: follow-up of fifty cases (abstr). The XVth World Federation of Hemophilia Congress, Stockholm, Sweden

Fonio A, Bühler W (1952) Die röntgenologische Darstellung des Blutergelenkes an Hand von 136 Gelenkaufnahme der Fonio'schen Sammlung. Radiol Clin 21: 316–322

Forbes CD, Greig WR, Prentice RM, McNicol GP (1972) Radioisotope knee joint scans in haemophilia and Christmas disease. J Bone Joint Surg [Br] 54: 468–475

Forrai J (1979) Radiology of haemophilic arthropathies. Martinus Nijhoff, The Hague Boston London

Ghadially FN, Roy S (1967) Histochemistry of synovium in experimental haemarthrosis in the rabbit. Ann Rheum Dis 26: 117–122

Gilbert MS (1977) Musculoskeletal manifestations of hemophilia. Mt Sinai J Med 44: 339–358

Harris ED Jr, Evanson JM, Dibone DR, Krang SM (1970) Collagenese and rheumatoid arthritis. Arthritis Rheum 13: 83–94

Heijnen L, de Groot C, Prevo A, Veltkamp J, Sjamsoedin-Visser L, Breederfeld C, Aronstam A (1983) Arthropathy in hemophiliacs, comparing long-term prophylaxis with treatment on demand. The XVth World Federation of Hemophilia Congress, Stockholm, Sweden

Heim M, Horoszowski H, Martinowitz U, Seligsohn U, Engel J (1982) Haemophiliac hands—a three year follow-up study. Hand 14: 333–336

Hilgartner MW, Arnold WD, Granda JL (1972) Acid phosphatase levels in synovial tissue fluid in patients with hemophilia. In: Proceedings of XIV International Congress of Hematology, Sao Paulo

Hoaglund F (1967) Experimental hemarthrosis, the response of canine knees to injections of autologous blood. J Bone Joint Surg [Am] 49: 285–298

Hough A, Banfield W, Sokoloff L (1976) Cartilage in hemophilic arthropathy: Ultrastructural and microanalytical studies. Arch Pathol Lab Med 100: 91–96

Johnson JB, Davis TW, Bullock WH (1954) Bone and joint changes in hemophilia. Radiology 63: 64–71

Jordan HH (1958) Hemophilic arthropathies. Charles C Thomas, Springfield, Ill

Key JA (1932) Hemophilic arthritis. Ann Surg 95: 198–225

Kingma MJ (1965) Overgrowth in hemophilia. Clin Orthop 39: 199–204

König F (1892) Die Gelenkerkrankungen bei Blutern mit besonderer Berücksichtigung der Diagnose. Klin Vorträge NF 36: 233–243. Translated in Clin Orthop 52: 5–11, 1967

Legg JW (1872) A treatise on haemophilia. Lewis, London

Leroux JL, Blotman F, Navarro N, Donnadio D, Izarn P, Simon L (1982) L'articulation fémuro-patellaire hémophilique. Rev Rhum Mal Osteoartic 49: 519–524

Levine PH (1974) Efficacy of self therapy in hemophilia. New Engl J Med 291: 1381–1384

Lewis JE, Sampson WI (1972) PTC deficiency with phalangeal and interphalangeal (arthritic) changes. Calif Med 116: 81–85

Licata G, Perricone R, Scaglione R (1977) L'artropatia emofilica indagata con fotoscintigrafia con ^{99m}Tc. Reumatismo 29: 83–87

Longmaid HE, Weissman BN (1982) Resorptive hip arthropathy in hemophilia. J Can Assoc Radiol 33: 43–45

Maquet PGJ (1976) Biomechanics of the knee. Springer, New York

Moseley JE (1963) Bone changes in haematologic disorders (roentgen aspects). Grune and Stratton, New York London

Nilsson IM, Hedner U, Ahlberg Å, Pettersson H, Noréhn K (1981) Current situations of prophylaxis and home infusion in Sweden. Proc 2nd Int Symp Hemophilia Treatm, pp 65–71

Otto J (1803) An account of an hemorrhagic disposition existing in certain families. Medial Repository 6: 1

Pavlov H, Foldman AB, Arnold WD (1979) Haemophilic arthropathy in the joints of the hands and feet. Br J Radiol 52: 173–180

Perry G (1978) Widening of the radial notch of the ulna: a new articular change in haemophilia. Clin Radiol 29: 61–62

Pettersson H, Nilsson IM (1982) Radiologic evaluation of the effect of prophylaxis. First International Workshop on Prevention in Hemophilia. Neve Ilan, Israel

Pettersson H, Nilsson IM (1984) Review of ongoing prophylaxis in Sweden. Second International Workshop on Prevention in Haemophilia. Paris, France

Pettersson H, Ahlberg Å, Nilsson IM (1980) A radiologic classification of hemophilic arthropathy. Clin Orthop 149: 153–159

Pettersson H, Nilsson IM, Hedner U, Noréhn K, Ahlberg Å (1981) Radiologic evaluation of prophylaxis in severe haemophilia. Acta Pediatr Scand 70: 565–570

Robinson HJ Jr, Granda JL (1974) Prostaglandins in synovial inflammatory disease. Surg Forum 25: 476–477

Rosner F (1969) Hemophilia in the Talmud and Rabbinic writings. Ann Intern Med 70: 833–837

Salerno NB, Menges JF, Borns PF (1972) Arthrograms in hemophilia. Radiology 102: 135–138

Schreiber RR (1975) Musculo-skeletal system—radiologic findings. In: Brinkhous KM, Hemker HC (eds) Handbook of hemophilia, part I. Excerpta Medica, Amsterdam, pp 333–370

Shaw JE (1897) A case of haemophilia with joint-lesion. Bristol Med Chir J 15: 240–244

Soeur R (1949) The synovial membrane of the knee in pathological conditions. J Bone Joint Surg [Am] 31: 317–340

Stoker DJ, Murray RO (1974) Skeletal changes in hemophilia and other bleeding disorders. Semin Roentgenol 9: 185–193

Storti E, Traldi A, Toscati E, Davoli P (1969) Synovectomy: A new approach to hemophilic arthropathy. Acta Haematol 41: 193–205

Swanton M (1959) Hemophilic arthropathy in dogs. Lab Invest 8: 1269–1277

Teitelbaum S (1977) Radiologic evaluation of the hemophilic hip. Mt Sinai J Med 44: 400–401

Trueta J (1963) Studies on the etiopathology of osteoarthritis of the hip. Clin Orthop 31: 7–19

van Creveld S, Kingma MJ (1961) Subperiosteal hemorrhage in hemophilia A and B. Acta Pediatr Scand 50: 291–296

van Creveld S, Hogdemaeker PJ, Kingma MJ, Wagenvoort CA (1971) Degeneration of joints in haemophiliacs under treatment by modern methods. J Bone Joint Surg [Br] 53: 296–302

Volkmann R (1868) Neue Beiträge zur Pathologie und Therapie der Krankenheit der Bewegungsorgane. A Hirschweld, Berlin

Winston ME (1952) Haemophilic arthropathy of the hip. J Bone Joint Surg [Br] 34: 412–420

Wolf CR, Mankin HJ (1965) The effect of experimental hemarthrosis on articular cartilage of rabbit knee joints. J Bone Joint Surg [Am] 47: 1203–1210

Wood K, Omer A, Shaw MT (1969) Haemophilic arthropathy. A combined radiological and clinical study. Br J Radiol 42: 498–505

Young JM, Hudacek MD (1954) Experimental production of pigmented villonodular synovitis in dogs. Am J Pathol 30: 799–811

Zimbler S, McVerry B, Levine P (1976) Hemophilic arthropathy of the foot and ankle. Orthop Clin North Am 7: 985–997

Chapter 4
Hemophilic Synovitis

A number of hemophilic patients will develop a persistent synovitis with swelling of a joint, and this condition appears to be inflammatory rather than hemorrhagic. This represents a poorly understood clinical syndrome. The natural history of such swelling is variable in that it may persist for months or years, may progress rapidly into a classic hemophilic arthropathy, or at times may clear spontaneously. It may be difficult to differentiate synovitis from recurrent bleeding, and at times there seems to be a close relationship between them. These two conditions represent what König (1892) referred to as the second-stage of hemophilic arthropathy. Because of the clinical importance of this condition, it will be described in some detail in this chapter.

Clinical Findings

Hemophilic synovitis is most common at the knee but may also be seen at the elbow and ankle. It is rarely diagnosed at other joints. It is most commonly seen between the ages of 6 and 16 years and is quite uncommon in the adult hemophiliac. The characteristic finding is a persistent effusion which is relatively painless. The effusion is usually quite large but not tense as in severe hemarthrosis. Tenderness is absent or minimal and there is the suggestion that there is an exuberant synovium within the joint in addition to the obvious fluid. A full range of motion is usually maintained in contrast to hemarthrosis, where spasm and marked limitation of motion are noted. Some capsular instability has been described. Characteristic of this condition is the lack of rapid response to factor replacement therapy.

Fluid aspirated from these joints is always blood tinged. The hematocrit will range from 8 to 35 (Gilbert 1977). Enzyme studies show increased levels of cathepsin D and acid phosphatase (Arnold and Hilgartner 1977). If such a joint is explored surgically, the synovium is noted to be exuberant and hypertrophic. It is stained dark-brown and usually fills most of the expanded joint cavity (Fig. 4.1). On microscopic evaluation, the fine fibrillar consistency of normal synovium is replaced by hypertrophic villi which are laden with hemosiderin. The synovium itself is very vascular, and perivascular infiltrates with inflammatory cells are noted.

The protean nature of the natural history of this condition has already been

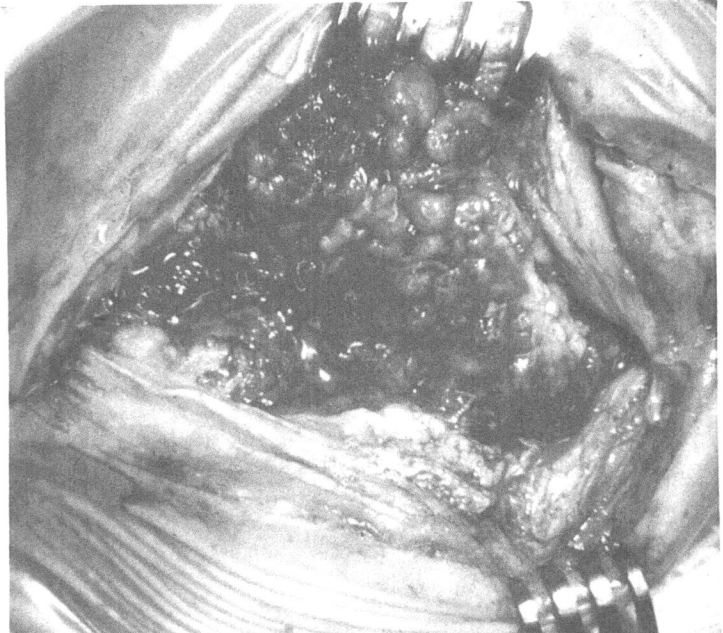

Fig. 4.1. Hypertrophic synovium as seen at surgical synovectomy.

referred to. The synovitis does respond dramatically to steroid therapy but it usually recurs upon discontinuation of the drug. Chemical synovectomy with osmic acid (Risse et al. 1973) or radioactive gold (Ahlberg 1973; Fernandez-Pallazi and de Bosch 1983) or even surgical synovectomy (Storti et al. 1970) may be required. If left untreated, the synovitis is followed by degenerative changes within the joint and a resultant stiff or painful joint may be seen.

Diagnostic Imaging

Radiologic evaluation of these joints does not show any characteristic bone changes but there is a pronounced increase in the density of the joint space and recesses, due either to the fluid or the hypertrophic synovium. At the knee the suprapatellar pouch, the joint cavity, and the popliteal swelling are best seen on a lateral radiograph (Fig. 4.2). At the ankle the swelling is noted anteriorly and posteriorly, again on a lateral radiograph (Fig. 4.3). In the elbow, synovitis is less easy to identify radiologically (Fig. 3.3). One of the characteristics that should be noted is that despite the significant effusion there may be little cartilage or bone involvement. We have noted that at the knee there is relatively more involvement of the patellofemoral compartment than at other compartments within the joint (Fig. 4.4). Axial views of the patella may help to evaluate these changes, and frequently lateral

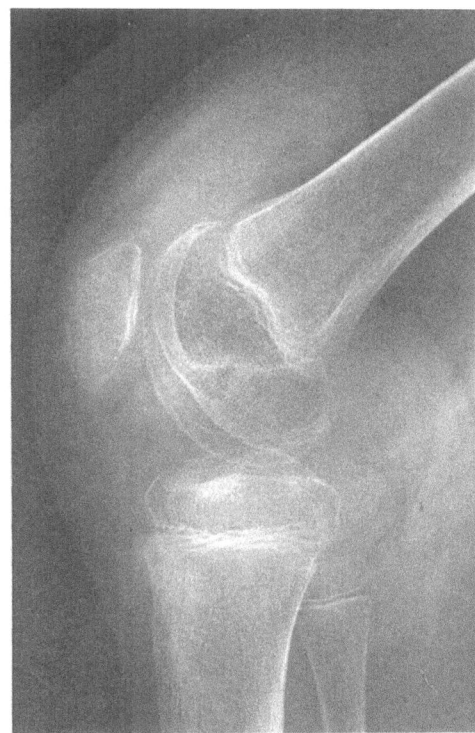

Fig. 4.2. Hemophilic synovitis at the knee. 12-year-old with severe hemophilia A. There is a pronounced bulging of the suprapatellar pouch and the popliteal area. The changes within the bone are moderate.

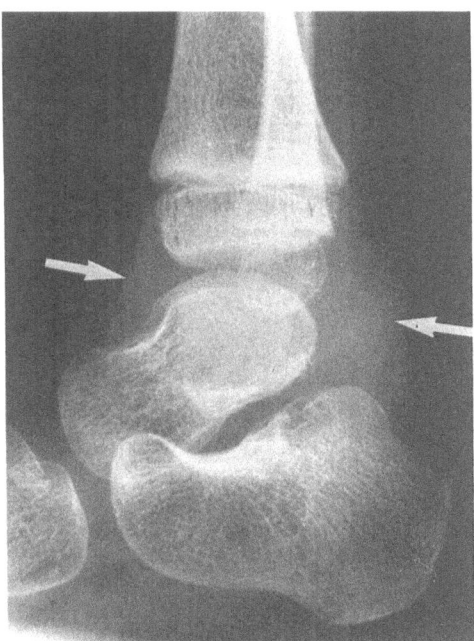

Fig. 4.3. Hemophilic synovitis at the ankle. 5-year-old with severe hemophilia A. The hypertrophic synovium is best seen anteriorly and posteriorly on the lateral view (*arrows*).

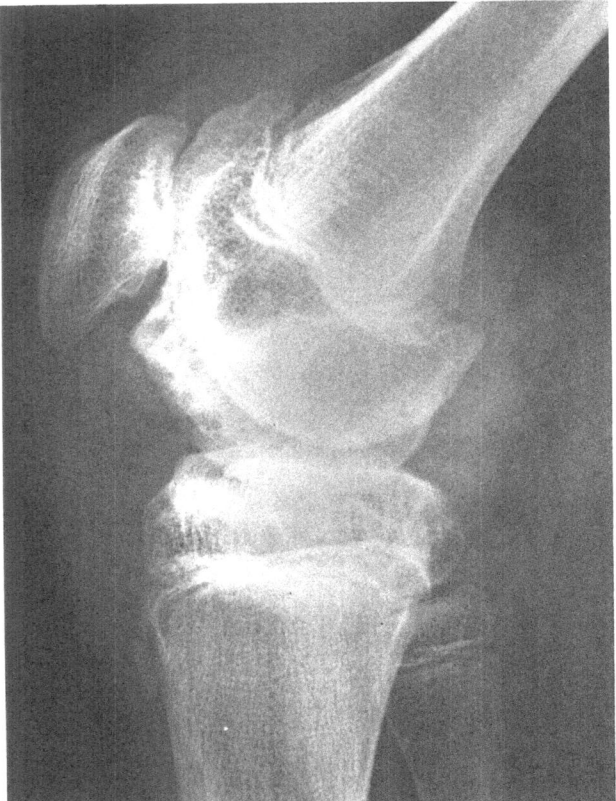

Fig. 4.4. Patellofemoral involvement in hemophilic synovitis. 13-year-old with severe hemophilia A. Severe skeletal changes at the patellofemoral compartment, and soft tissue changes consistent with synovitis. The changes at the tibiofemoral compartment are less pronounced.

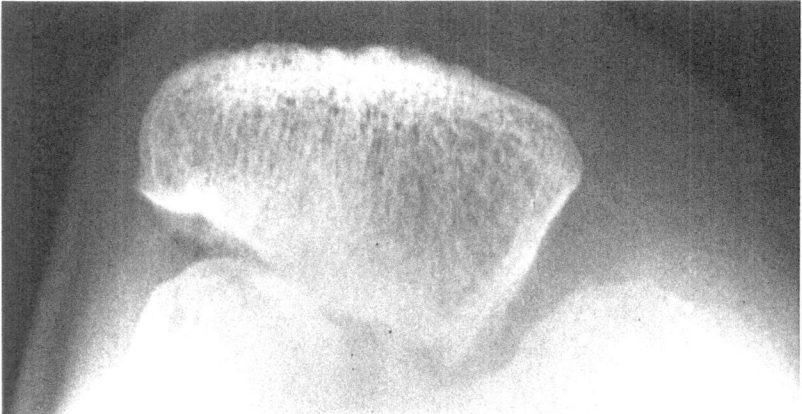

Fig. 4.5. Axial view of the patella in hemophilic synovitis. On this view the lateral positioning of the patella can be appreciated. Note the subchondral irregularity and narrowing of the cartilage.

subluxation of the patella is noted (Fig. 4.5). There is some debate as to whether patellofemoral degenerative changes and subluxation result in the synovitis or whether the capsular laxity frequently seen with this problem allows the lateral subluxation. Further evaluation of this problem is necessary.

Diagnostic imaging of this condition by other techniques has not been very rewarding. Double contrast arthrography has proven difficult to evaluate because of the exuberant synovium. Frequently the joint is loculated and only a small portion can be visualized by the contrast material (Schreiber 1975). Radioisotope imaging outlines the inflammatory nature of the process but is not clinically helpful. Ultrasonography may become useful in differentiating synovial hypertrophy from effusion.

References

Ahlberg Å (1973) Radioactive gold in treatment of chronic synovial effusion in haemophilia. In: Ala F, Denson KWE (eds) Haemophilia. Excerpta Medica, Amsterdam

Arnold WD, Hilgartner MW (1977) Hemophilic arthropathy: Current concepts of pathogenesis and management. J Bone Joint Surg [Am] 59: 287–305

Fernandez-Pallazi F, de Bosch NB (1983) Radioactive synoviorthesis in hemophilic hemarthrosis. Follow-up of fifty cases. The XVth World Federation of Hemophilia Congress, Stockholm, Sweden

Gilbert MS (1977) Musculoskeletal manifestation of hemophilia. Mt Sinai J Med 44: 339–358

König F (1892) Die Gelenkerkrankungen bei Blutern mit besonderer Berücksichtigung der Diagnose. Klin Vorträge NF 36: 233. Translated in Clin Orthop 52: 5–11, 1967

Risse JC, Menkes C, Allain JP, Witvoet J (1973) Synoviorthesis in the treatment of chronic haemophilic arthropathy: A preliminary report. In: Ala F, Denson KWE (eds) Haemophilia. Excerpta Medica, Amsterdam

Schreiber RR (1975) Musculo-skeletal system—radiologic findings. In: Brinkhous KM, Hemker HC (eds) Handbook of Hemophilia. Excerpta Medica, Amsterdam, pp 333–370

Storti E, Traldi E, Tosatti E, Davoli G (1970) Synovectomy in hemophilia: A new therapeutic approach and efficient technique of hemostasis. Gazetta Sanitaria 14: 11–17

Chapter 5

Soft Tissue Bleeding

Bleeding into the soft tissues is a common occurrence in the hemophilias. The clinical spectrum ranges from subcutaneous ecchymosis to intramuscular hematomas to compartment syndromes with subsequent neurovascular compromise. Because of this variability, it is difficult to estimate the incidence of many of these lesions. Almost all patients have bruises characterized by subcutaneous discoloration. In contrast to platelet disorders in which ecchymosis occurs spontaneously, these lesions usually follow trauma in hemophilia. The ecchymosis might be quite extensive but rarely requires treatment. It is the deep hematomas that are of greater concern. The extent of damage will depend upon the extent of hemorrhage and the containment provided by the various fascial compartments. Small hematomas in large muscle masses resorb without complication. Similar hematomas in tight fascial compartments may cause ischemic myopathy. Large hematomas, even in large muscle masses, may resorb slowly, and the resultant fibrosis may limit the excursion of the muscle and cause severe contracture.

Clinical Considerations

Favre-Gilly (1968) noted that 76% of his young hemophiliacs experienced one or more intramuscular bleeding episodes. In Duthie's series (1972) 70 of 457 bleeding episodes were intramuscular. Thus it appears that this is the second most common site of bleeding in hemophilia, following only intra-articular hemorrhage. There appears to be no predilection for either the upper or the lower extremities. Bleeding does occur into the muscles of the trunk but with a lesser frequency. In the upper extremity, bleeding occurs most commonly in the flexor muscles, but in the lower extremity it is most common at the quadriceps and calf.

Signs and Symptoms

Trauma may be a predisposing cause, but as with the hemarthrosis, bleeding may occur "spontaneously," perhaps due to the stresses of daily activity. Another cause of deep hematomas are intramuscular injections, which should be avoided in these bleeding diatheses.

The symptoms vary considerably and lack of early recognition may lead to delay in treatment. Pain, while a prominent symptom, may not be severe and may not be manifest until late. Swelling is not appreciated at first as this may be deep within the soft tissues. The pain and swelling is determined by the fascial confines of the affected muscles. As noted before, symptoms will be more acute in areas where there is limited space for distention. Limitation of motion and spasm without evidence of a hemarthrosis should lead to suspicion of an intramuscular hemorrhage. Tenderness and induration secondary to the inflammatory response will follow.

Pathology

The pathology has been well described by Duthie (1972). He noted that the bleeding occurs within the substance of the muscle. Muscle fibers, surrounded by blood, die and avascular structures are seen imbedded within the clots. The cellular response includes an exudation of polymorphonuclear leukocytes, phagocytic mononuclear cells, and the appearance of immature connective tissue cells. Resorption of clots and necrotic muscle is followed by fibrosis. Duthie noted that "there is no effective regeneration of muscle fibers following large hematomas." Maturation of the collagenous fibrous tissue produces contracture and may lead to further damage of the muscle cells. Muscle fibers enmeshed in this fibrous tissue will become atrophic and show degenerative changes such as central migration of sarcolemmal nuclei.

Sequelae

Most intramuscular hematomas resolve without clinical sequelae, but significant complications such as contracture, neuropathy, and pseudotumor formation must be of concern.

Contracture

Favre-Gilly (1968) and Duthie (1972) noted that 10% and 11% respectively of muscle hematomas were followed by a permanent contracture. The most common sites of permanent contracture are at the calf and forearm. Therefore equinus deformity at the foot and ankle and flexion deformity at the wrist and hand are not uncommon. The latter is frequently associated with neurologic involvement. Hip flexion deformity following iliopsoas hemorrhage occurs, but bleeding at the shoulder, buttock, and quadriceps usually resolves without permanent loss of motion. Since trauma with resultant hemorrhage and muscle necrosis have been implicated as factors predisposing to myositis ossificans, one might assume that this would occur frequently in hemophilia. However, it is rarely reported (Schreiber 1975; Lancourt et al. 1977). Similarly, peripheral vascular compromise is rare. Reports of gangrene (Biggs and Matthews 1966) are unusual and almost all were noted prior to the availability of factor replacement.

Peripheral Neuropathy

Peripheral nerve involvement is common in hemophilia and is usually the result of intramuscular bleeding. In 1964 Silverstein at the Mount Sinai Hospital in New York found 31 peripheral nerve lesions in 206 patients. Gendelman (1977) at the same institution followed 201 patients from 1964 until 1977 and reported that 26 had involvement of the peripheral nervous system. At Oxford 23 of 113 patients followed from 1966 to 1969 had 29 peripheral nerve lesions. Both Duthie (1972) and Gilchrist et al. (1982) pointed out that almost all of these occurred in adults and that the lesions were rare in children. Alagille et al. (1966) noted a 10% incidence in a study of 117 children.

Gilchrist has pointed out that the most commonly affected nerve is the femoral nerve and that this is associated with the syndrome of iliopsoas hemorrhage. Bleeding in the forearm frequently results in median and ulnar nerve involvement. Sciatic involvement following intramuscular injection into the buttock has been seen. All other nerves can be involved, but with lesser frequency. It is a bit surprising that the ulnar nerve is often spared despite significant pathology at the elbow. Perhaps the slow development of this pathology accounts for this finding. We have noted only one case of an isolated ulnar nerve lesion and that was associated with a large synovial cyst within the ulnar groove. Several patients with complete dislocation secondary to hemophilic arthropathy have been followed without any evidence of a tardy ulnar paresis. Neuropathy associated with pseudotumor formation is not uncommon (Gilbert et al. 1982). Acute entrapment syndromes, such as carpal tunnel syndrome, have been reported. Intraneural bleeding has not been documented.

Pseudotumor Formation

The relationship of intramuscular hemorrhage to pseudotumor formation remains unclear. There is little question that in the adult, pseudotumors occur with highest frequency in the iliopsoas, the quadriceps, and the gastrocnemius muscle, common areas of intramuscular hemorrhage. Duthie (1972) has reported that "large accumulations of blood in muscle occasionally are too large for phagocytic cells to remove before the process of fibrosis has led to encapsulation and sealing off from surrounding viable tissue. When this occurs, the hematoma persists as a cystic lesion containing inspissated blood clots with altered hemoglobin and lipid material. Such cysts once formed may be expected to persist." The site of bleeding and its proximity to bone may also be an important factor. There are no good data to determine the exact relationship.

There is little question that large soft tissue hematomas must be followed to complete resorption to rule out transformation to pseudotumors. The initial size of large hematomas should be documented by ultrasonography and the resolution followed by serial studies. If resolution slows down or if complete obliteration of the cavity is not seen, a CT examination should be obtained. A hematoma may be differentiated from a pseudotumor in that the latter has a fibrous wall surrounding the central clot, as will be discussed below. If this is noted, surgical excision should be considered. The pseudotumor will be discussed in more detail in the next chapter.

Specific Sites of Involvement

Iliopsoas Muscle

The iliopsoas muscle is the most common site of intramuscular hemorrhage in hemophilia. Goodfellow et al. (1967) in a classic article explained the clinical syndrome by anatomic dissections with injection studies. They showed that the initial site of hemorrhage is the iliacus muscle, with secondary involvement of the psoas.

Pain in the groin with radiation to the back or thigh is the usual presenting symptom. The onset may be quite insidious. Trauma is not a common predisposing cause. The hip is held flexed and pain is noted on forced extension. Gentle rotation is not painful and this differentiates the syndrome from a hemarthrosis of the hip, which is rare. Swelling is noted at the iliac fossa, and abdominal guarding may mimic the finding of appendicitis. Goodfellow et al. (1967) noted a femoral palsy in all but one of their cases, but Duthie (1972) noted it in 12 of 19 cases. The iliacus hematoma is within a tight fascial compartment and the blood is forced distally to compress the femoral nerve. Bleeding into the psoas sheath usually tracks proximally and therefore is not associated with a femoral neuropathy. The clinical manifestations of this neuropathy include diminution of the patellar reflex, quadriceps weakness or paralysis, and loss of sensation over the anterior thigh. Despite early treatment of this syndrome, complete resolution of the neuropathy cannot be guaranteed. If quadriceps weakness persists, the knee is at risk of recurrent hemorrhage because of the trauma associated with repeated buckling.

Gastrocnemius Muscle

The calf is the second most common site of intramuscular hemorrhage but due to the lack of tight fascial containment, neuropathy is not common. However, there is a high incidence of persistent contracture, and equinus deformity may result. Pseudotumor formation in this area is also of concern.

Forearm

Bleeding into the forearm is a true emergency because of the tight compartmentalization and the importance of the structures running within these compartments. The anterior compartment is not an uncommon site of bleeding and if not treated promptly, ischemic fibrous contracture of the muscles and neuropathy of the ulnar and median nerves can result. Lancourt et al. (1977) reported this in six patients followed at Mount Sinai Hospital from 1969 to 1976. However, it should be noted that all of these lesions occurred before the availability of concentrated factor replacement, or in patients with inhibitors. Pseudotumors in this area are rare and this may be due to the fact that large hematomas cannot develop.

Diagnostic Imaging

The Hemorrhage and Its Resolution

Before the modern era of diagnostic imaging it was seldom possible to visualize the early stages of an intramuscular hematoma. However, with a large iliopsoas hematoma, the psoas shadow on the abdominal plain film is blurred out. The hematoma may also dislocate the ureter and bladder, which is demonstrable on an intravenous urogram (Fig. 5.1) (von Grauthoff et al. 1978; Heim et al. 1982). Intramuscular hematomas in the psoas muscle and elsewhere have also been demonstrated by blood pool scanning using TC^{99m} (Green et al. 1981).

Today, the diagnostic modalities of choice for imaging of fresh as well as resolving intramuscular hematomas are ultrasonography and computed tomography.

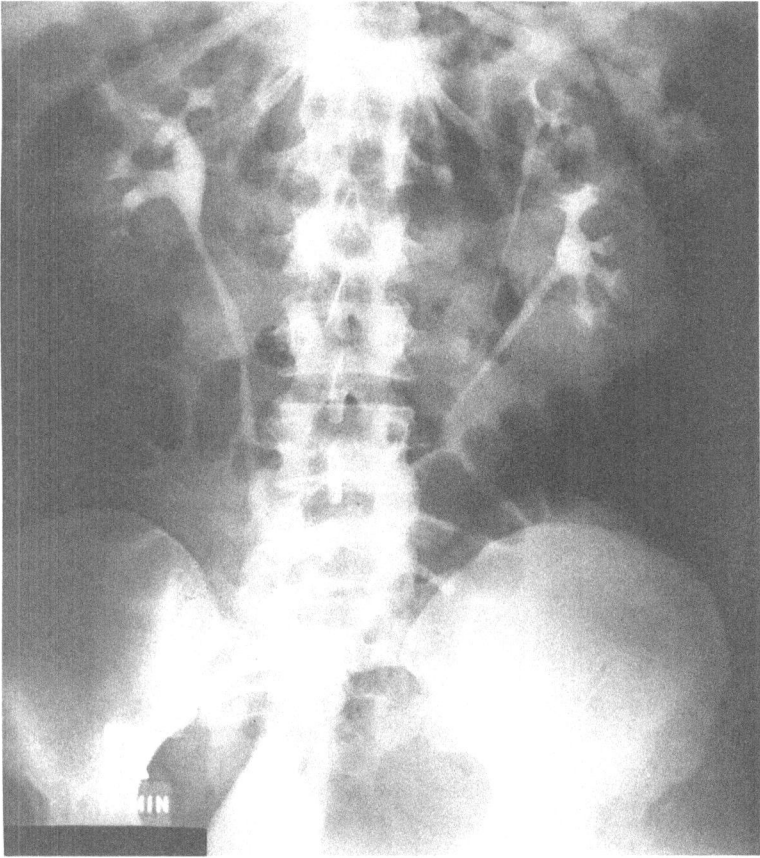

Fig. 5.1. Large iliopsoas hematoma, intravenous urography. 35-year-old with severe hemophilia B. The left ureter is stretched and dislocated towards the midline, and the bladder is dislocated and impressed from the left. The duplication of the left ureter is an incidental finding.

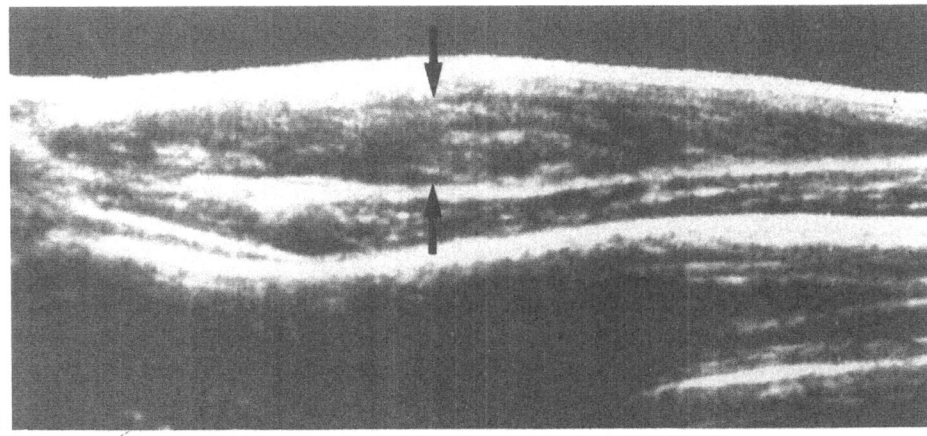

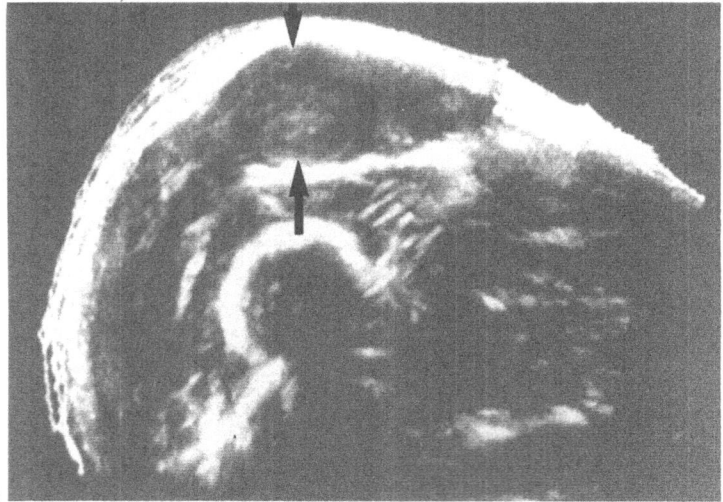

Fig. 5.2a,b. Hematoma of the rectus femoris muscle, ultrasonography. **a** longitudinal and **b** transverse section. There is an increase in the size of the muscle, with dislocation of the fascial planes and the muscle fibers (*arrows*). The hematoma is of complex type with hyperechoic and unechoic areas, indicating blood clot formation within the fluid.

Ultrasonography

On ultrasonography, the muscle in the early stage of bleeding may appear enlarged and more rounded as compared with the normal, contralateral side. At this stage it may not be possible to separate the hematoma from the muscle mass (Kumari et al. 1979; Wallis et al. 1981) (Fig. 5.2) and it may also be difficult to differentiate from an edema in the muscle. However, as a result of interstitial bleeding with dislocation of the muscle fibers, there is often an exaggeration of the "penniform" structure of the muscle (Fig. 5.3) (Aspelin et al. 1984). If the bleeding is a localized circumscribed lesion it is more easily detected by ultrasonography (Fig. 5.4). The bleeding itself may appear as an unechoic lesion with increased enhancement of

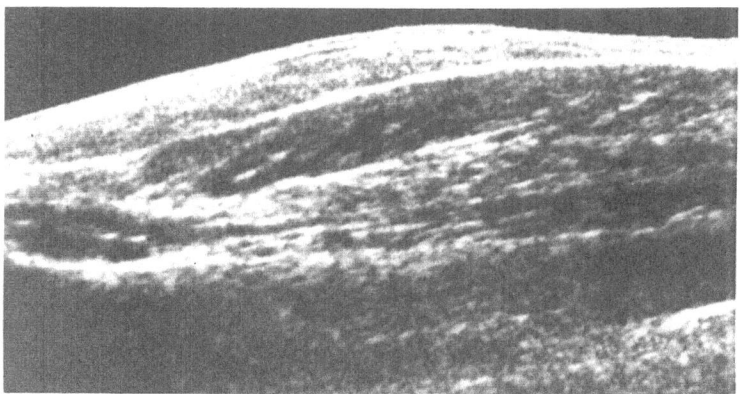

Fig. 5.3. Hematoma in the vastus medialis muscle, ultrasonography. Longitudinal section. The muscle is enlarged, with a pronounced "penniform structure," indicating diffuse bleeding.

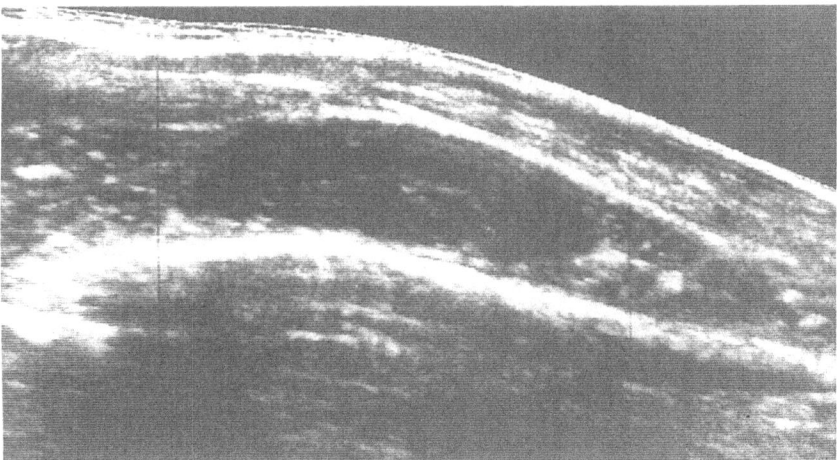

Fig. 5.4. Localized circumscribed unechoic hematoma in the vastus intermedius muscle, ultrasonography. Longitudinal section.

the echoes behind the lesion, indicating fluid (Fig. 5.5) and this appearance may later change into a more complex type with regions of hyperechoic structures within the fluid, indicating blood clot formation (Fig. 5.2) (Heim et al. 1982; Shirkoda et al. 1983; Wicks et al. 1978). In the later serous phase large hematomas may become unechoic again, because of liquefaction (Conte et al. 1982; Wicks et al. 1978).

If adequate factor replacement therapy is given, and the hematoma is of moderate size, the muscle returns to normal appearance as the hematoma resolves. This resolution may be rapid, being complete within 1–3 weeks (Aspelin et al. 1984), although other authors have reported considerably longer times for resolution of hemophilic muscle hematomas (Forbes et al. 1977; McVerry et al. 1977; Wicks et al. 1978).

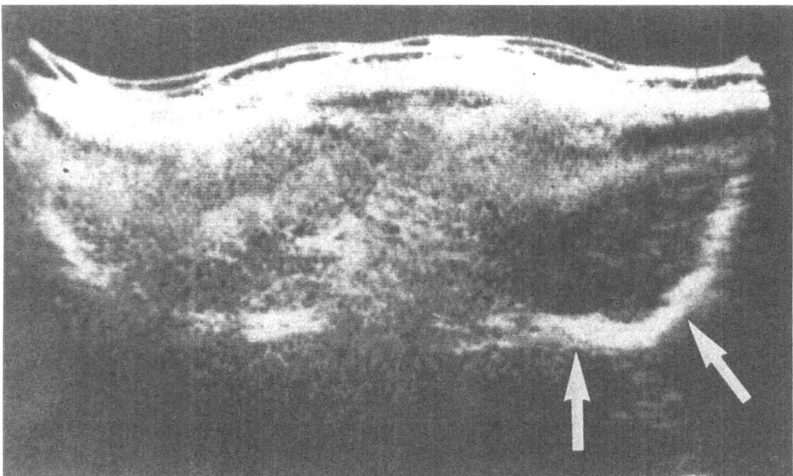

Fig. 5.5. Hematoma of the iliopsoas muscle, ultrasonography. Transverse section. There is an unechoic well defined lesion, with increased enhancement of the echoes behind the lesion (*arrows*) indicating fluid.

Computed Tomography

Using CT the delineation of the hematoma is more accurate, and the different stages of the hemorrhage are easier to define (Shirkoda et al. 1983). In the early stages, the fresh clotted blood has a high attenuation value, giving the lesion an inhomogeneous appearance (Fig. 5.6). During the resolution, this attenuation value diminishes, approaching that of normal muscle (Fig. 5.7) (van Lackner et al. 1978), and if the hematoma has liquefied, CT reveals a circumscribed area of low attenuation that may be surrounded by a capsule within the muscle (Fig. 5.8) (von Lackner et al. 1978). If such a capsule is seen, the development of a pseudotumor must be suspected. The patient must be followed with repeat CT examination and surgery might be considered. Although the CT examination gives a more detailed view of the intramuscular hemorrhage, the ultrasonographic examination provides all necessary information, not only for diagnosis but also for follow-up during treatment (McVerry et al. 1977). Being a safe method giving no ionizing radiation, ultrasonography should be the method of choice in these cases (Aspelin et al. 1984).

Magnetic Resonance Imaging

In the future, MRI may give detailed additional information about the hematoma itself as well as tissue changes caused by the bleeding. Figure 5.9 shows a soft tissue hemorrhage in the calf, as appearing in MRI.

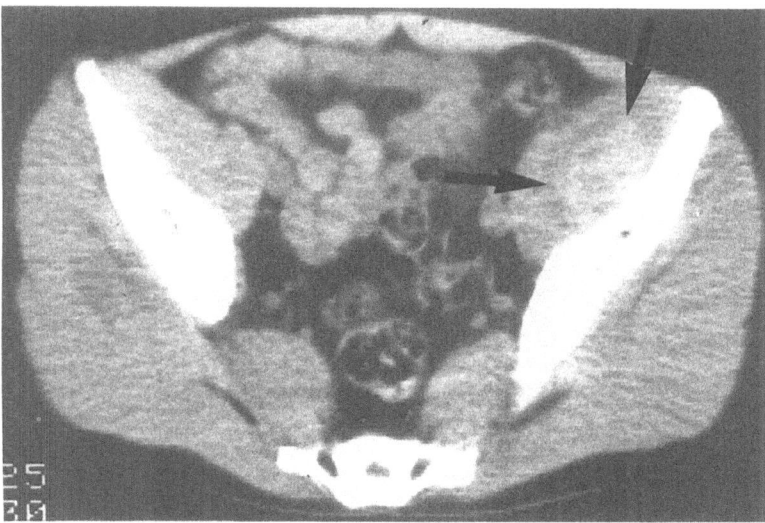

Fig. 5.6. Fresh iliopsoas hematoma, CT. 16-year-old with severe hemophilia A. The left iliopsoas muscle is enlarged owing to a lesion with inhomogeneous attenuation (*arrows*), indicating fresh bleeding with a mixture of liquid blood and blood clots.

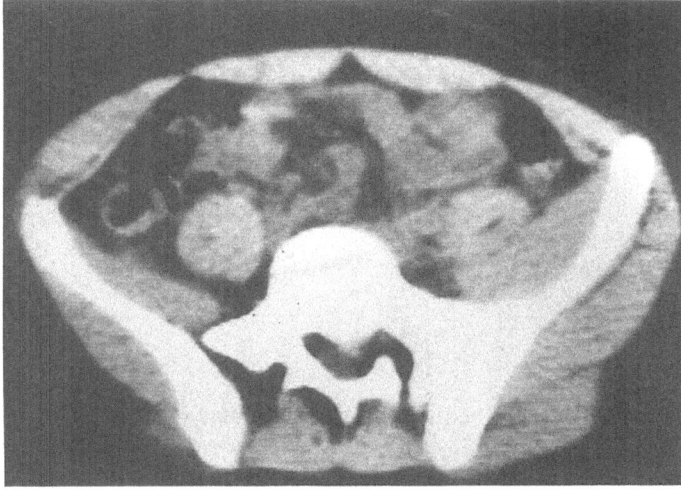

Fig. 5.7. Resolving iliopsoas hematoma, CT. 20-year-old with severe hemophilia A. After 3 weeks of factor replacement therapy for an iliopsoas hematoma, the left muscle is larger than the normal right muscle, but the attenuation values of the muscles are the same.

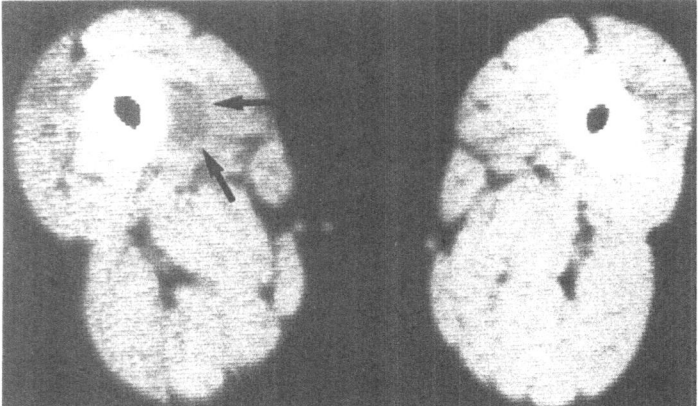

Fig. 5.8. Liquefied hematoma, CT. 24-year-old with severe hemophilia A. In the right thigh, close to the femur, there is a circumscribed area of low attenuation, surrounded by a capsule (*arrows*). This must be suspected to be the first sign of pseudotumor formation.

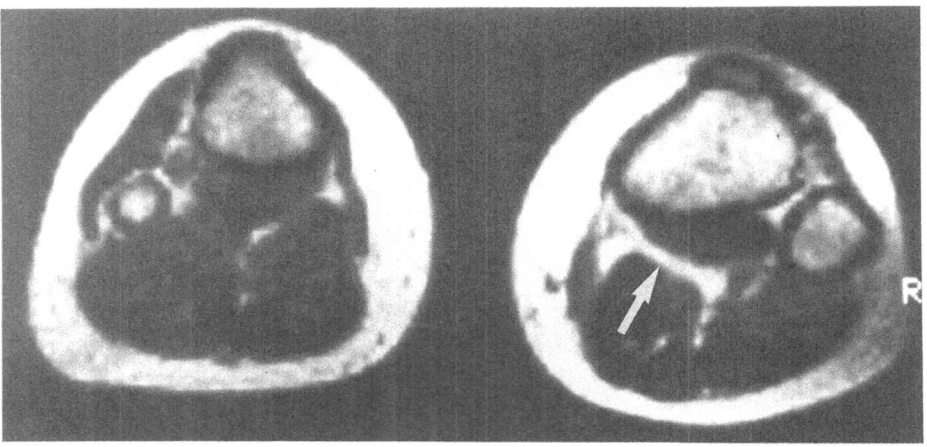

Fig. 5.9. Soft tissue hemorrhage in the calf, MRI. Severe hemophilia A. This T2-weighted image is obtained with a Diasonics MT/S system, using a supraconducting magnet operating at 3.5 K Gauss. The signal from the static extravasated blood has a high intensity (*arrow*). (By courtesy of Hans Ringertz, MD, Department of Radiology, UCSF Medical School, San Francisco, U.S.A.)

Sequelae

Heterotopic new bone formation as a sequela of intramuscular hemorrhage may be seen in its early stage in CT examinations (von Lackner et al. 1978) and later on plain film radiography. Probably because of its limited clinical significance such myositis ossificans in hemophilia has been documented only scantily in the radiologic literature (Heim et al. 1979; Hutcheson 1973; Petersen 1947; Sampinato 1970; Vas et al. 1981)..

In nearly all cases of myositis ossificans in hemophilia, trauma has preceded the muscle damage and hemorrhage (Vas et al. 1981). One explanation of the new bone formation may be that the hematomas have been situated close to the bone, generating periosteal osteoblastic activity (Fig. 5.10). Such periosteal reaction may arise also in the fascia between muscle groups. However, heterotopic new bone formation may also appear in hemorrhage far from the skeleton (Fig. 5.11), and in these cases there is probably metaplasia of the connective tissue, developed during the healing process (Vas et al. 1981).

In all reports, a peripelvic location is most common, and a large piece of bone extending between the ischial tuberosity and the lesser trochanter has been described by most authors (Heim et al. 1979; Hutcheson 1973; Vas et al. 1981). This ossification in the proximal part of the adductor magnus muscle may be characteristic for hemophilia (Fig. 5.12) (Vas et al. 1981). Many other sites have been described, for instance around the knee, in the extraspinal region, and the thigh musculature (Fig. 5.13) (Vas et al. 1981).

Peripheral nerve involvement is a well recognized complication, as discussed above in this chapter. The dislocation of the femoral nerve caused by the hematoma has been visualized on ultrasound (Heim et al. 1982) and should be possible to detect on CT examination.

Hemophilic pseudotumor is discussed in Chap. 6.

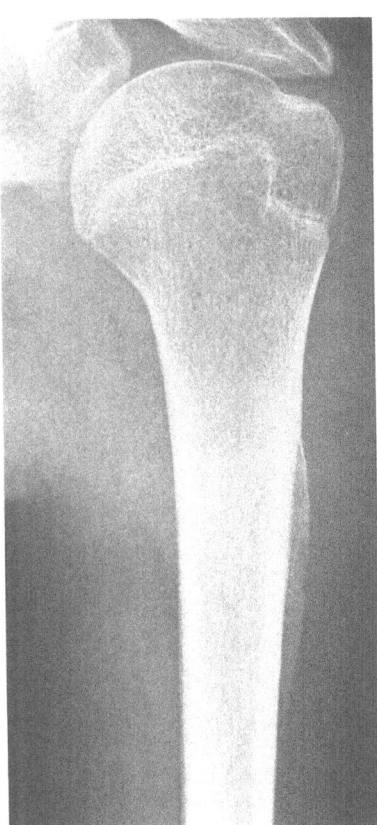

Fig. 5.10. Heterotopic new bone formation. 16-year-old with severe hemophilia A. Six months after a hematoma in the upper arm there is new bone formation close to the humerus, probably caused by a periosteal reaction.

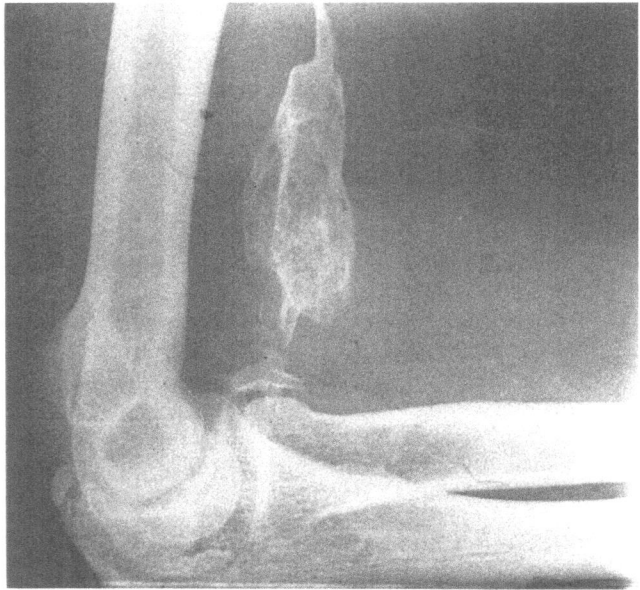

Fig. 5.11. Heterotopic new bone formation in the soft tissues of the elbow. 20-year-old with severe hemophilia A.

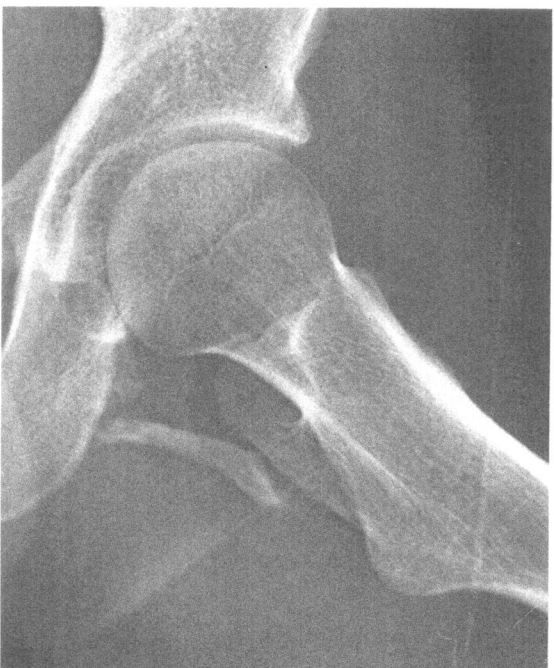

Fig. 5.12. Heterotopic new bone formation extending between the ischial tuberosity and the trochanter. 18-year-old with severe hemophilia B. This ossification in the adductor magnus muscle may be characteristic for hemophilic heterotopic new bone formation.

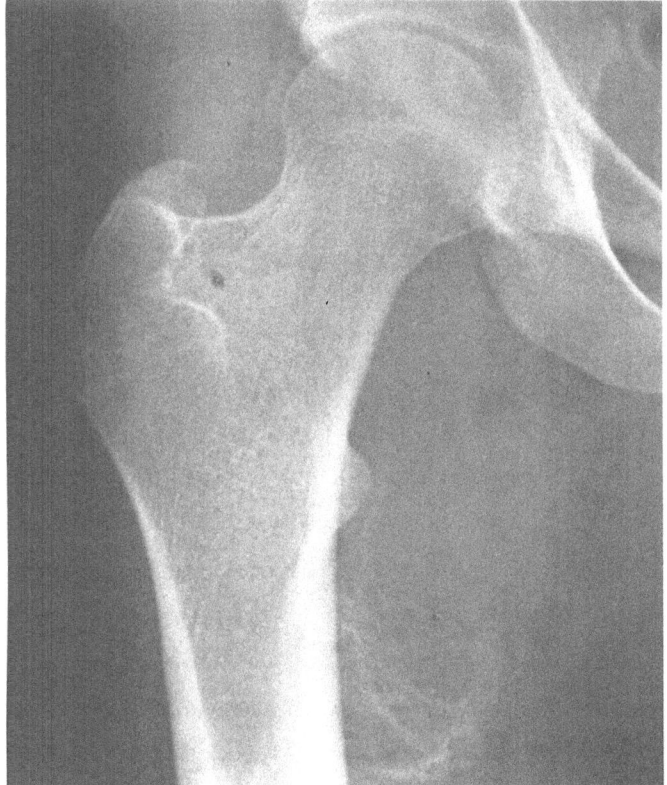

Fig. 5.13. Heterotopic new bone formation in the thigh. 25-year-old with severe hemophilia B.

References

Alagille J, Josso F, Queneau P (1966) Les accidents neurologiques peripheriques chez l'enfant hémophie. Arch Fr Pediatr 23: 819–838

Aspelin P, Pettersson H, Sigurjonsson S, Nilsson IM (1984) Ultrasonographic examinations of muscle hematomas in hemophiliacs. Acta Radiologica 25: 513–516

Biggs R, Matthews JM (1966) The treatment of spontaneous bleeding in haemophilia. In: Biggs R, MacFarlane RG (eds) Treatment of haemophilia and other coagulation disorders. Blackwell, Oxford

Conte G, Avelar F, Pizzuto J, Aviles A, Ambriz y Armando Sinco R (1982) Ultrasonographia en el diagnostico del hematoma retroperitoneal en el paciente hemofilico. Rev Med Chile 110: 255–262

Duthie RB, Matthews JM, Rizza CR, Stel VM (1972) The management of musculo-skeletal problems in the haemophilias. Blackwell Scientific, Oxford

Favre-Gilly J (1968) Expérience de cinq ans du centre Emile Remigny de Montain (Jura) pour jeunes garcons hémophiles. Hemostase 4: 231

Forbes CD, Lowe GDU, Prentice CRM (1977) Ultrasonography in hemophilia. Lancet I: 1064–1065

Gendelman S (1977): Hemophilia and the nervous system. Mt Sinai J Med 44: 402–408

Gilbert MS, Kreel I, Hermann G (1982): The hemophilic pseudotumor. In: Hilgartner MW (ed) Hemophilia in the child and adult. Masson, New York

Gilchrist GS, Piepgras DG, Ruskos RR (1982) Neurologic complications in hemophilia. In: Hilgartner MW (ed) Hemophilia in the child and adult. Masson, New York

Goodfellow J, Fearn CB D'A, Matthews JM (1967) Iliacus haematoma—a common complication of haemophilia. J Bone Joint Surg [Br] 49: 748–756

Green D, Spies SM, Rana NA, Milgram JW, Mintzer R (1981) Hemophilic bleeding evaluated by blood pool scanning. Thromb Haemost 45: 208–210

Heim M, Horoszowski H, Seligson U, Martinowitz U, Strauss S (1982) Ilio-psoas hematoma—its detection and treatment, with special reference to hemophilia. Arch Orthop Trauma Surg 99: 195–197

Hutcheson J (1973) Peripelvic new bone formation in hemophilia. Report of three cases. Diagn Radiol 109: 529–530

Kumari S, Fulco J, Karayalcin G, Lipton R (1979) Gray scale ultrasound: Evaluation of iliopsoas hematomas in hemophiliacs. AJR 133: 103–106

Lancourt JE, Gilbert MS, Posner MA (1977) Management of bleeding and associated complications of hemophilia in the hand and forearm. J Bone Joint Surg [Am] 59: 451–460

McVerry BA, Voke J, Vicary FR, Dormandy KM (1077) Ultrasonography in the management of hemophilia. Lancet I: 872–874

Petersen J (1947) A case of osseous changes in a patient with hemophilia. Acta Radiol 28: 323–330

Sampinato F (1970) Ossificaziono modellate nelle parti moli in soggetti emofilici. Rev Radiol 10: 52–61

Schreiber RR (1975) Musculo-skeletal system. Radiologic findings. In: Brinkhous KB, Hemker MC (eds) Handbook of hemophilia. Excerpta Medica, Amsterdam

Shirkoda A, Mauro MA, Staab EV, Blatt PM (1982) Soft-tissue haemorrhage in hemophiliac patients. Computed tomography and ultrasound study. Radiology 147: 811–814

Silverstein A (1964) Management of neurologic complications of hemophilia. In: Brinkhous KM (ed) The hemophilias. University of North Carolina Press, Chapel Hill

Vas W, Cockshott WP, Martin RF, Pai MK, Walker I (1981) Myositis ossificans in hemophilia. Skeletal Radiol 7: 27–31

von Grauthoff H, Hofmann P, Lackner K, Brackmann HH (1978) Hämophiler Pseudotumor und Ilia-cushämatom; radiologische und klinische Befunde. RÖFO 129: 614–620

von Lackner K, Hofmann P, Grauthoff H, Brecht G, Thurn P (1978) Computertomographischer Nachweis von Muskelhämatomen bei Hämophilie. RÖFO 129: 298–302

Wallis J, van Kaick G, Schimpf K, Zeltsch P (1981) Ultrasound diagnosis of muscle haematomas in hemophiliac patients (authors' transl). RÖFO 134: 153–156

Wicks JD, Silver TM, Bree RL (1978) Gray scale features of hematomas: An ultrasonic spectrum. Am J Roentgenol 131: 977–980

Chapter 6

The Hemophilic Pseudotumor

The pseudotumor is the most spectacular and serious of all the musculoskeletal lesions seen in hemophilia. It was first described, in the German literature, by Starker in 1918. Since then over one hundred cases have been reported. In a review of his experience at Oxford, Gunning (1966) estimated its incidence to be about 1% of all severe hemophiliacs. Most of these cases occurred before the advent of adequate factor replacement, and Gilbert stated in 1975 that "with improved treatment its incidence appears to be on the wane." However, despite the availability of early factor replacement the elimination of this entity has not been achieved, a fair number of new lesions being seen each year. The natural history and clinical and radiologic manifestations have been well documented, but etiologic factors such as the original site of hemorrhage and the factors that lead to encapsulation rather than resorption remain obscure.

Early diagnosis should be the aim of the radiologist. The diagnosis should be made before the more severe manifestations such as neuropathy or bone destruction become evident.

Definition

de Valderrama and Matthews in 1965 characterized the pseudotumor as "a progressive cystic swelling involving muscle, produced by recurrent hemorrhage, and accompanied by radiographic evidence of bone involvement." They classified hemophilic cysts into three categories:

"1. The simple cyst which occurs within the fascial envelope of a muscle or muscles and which is confined by the tendinous attachments.

2. The cyst which develops in a muscle with wide fibrous periosteal attachments and which may progress to give rise to cortical thinning because it interferes with the periosteal blood supply.

3. The pseudotumor which starts as a subperiosteal hemorrhage with stripping of the periosteum from the cortex until this is limited by aponeurotic or tendinous attachments and which then raises or destroys the muscles."

They felt that these represented different entities, but it is our feeling that they represent three different stages of the same entity, in which the amount of soft tissue and bone destruction are dependent upon the original site of hemorrhage and anatomic variation.

Ahlberg (1975), Gilbert (1975), and Martinson (1976) independently concluded that the clinical patterns of pseudotumor formation in the mature and immature skeleton were different, and they will be treated as two different entities in this chapter. However, it should be kept in mind that although the different patterns seem to suggest different etiologies, the distinction is not always sharp and our poor basic understanding of pseudotumors does not allow a clear picture to be drawn of the basic etiology and pathology.

The Adult

Clinical Considerations

Because many of the pseudotumors recorded in the literature occurred before the advent of replacement therapy, we can trace the natural history of this entity. The patient usually presents with an expanding painless mass in the area of the pelvis, thigh, or leg. Lesions in the upper extremity are rare in the adult, as are those in the hand and foot. The sites of pseudotumors treated at Mount Sinai Hospital, New York, are noted in Table 6.1. The mass is usually firm, nontender, and adherent to the deep structures. The singular lack of symptomatology may account for the fact that unless the patient is routinely followed by a physician, it may be years before he seeks medical attention for this problem. In the literature there was an average delay of 8 years before consulting a physician (Gilbert 1975). A prior history of trauma is common in lesions of the limbs, and the patient frequently recalls a significant hematoma which either resolved slowly or not at all. A history of trauma is rare in pseudotumors of the pelvis, but many patients can recall a history of bleeding "about the hip." After the initial response to bleeding, a mass may persist which may enlarge at irregular intervals. Arteriovascular compromise is rare, but some evidence of venous stasis may arise.

Progressive enlargement may result in neuropathy. Femoral nerve entrapment is not uncommon in pelvic or proximal femoral pseudotumors, but sciatic and more peripheral neuropathies have also been noted. Progressive bone destruction of the

Table 6.1. Hemophilic pseudotumors, Mt. Sinai Hospital 1969–1984

Site	No.
Pelvis	6
Buttock	2
Thigh	6
Leg	3
Back	1
Heel	1
	19 (16 patients)

femur and tibia may result in pathologic fracture. Rapid enlargement of the pseudotumor associated with the onset of pain should signal this possibility. Rarely the pseudotumor may enlarge enough to compromise the overlying skin. Prior to factor replacement this complication was usually followed by sinus formation, infection, septicemia, and death. Iliac pseudotumors have been reported to erode into the bowel with exsanguination. However, despite these ominous complications other pseudotumors may remain static for years. At present we know of no prognostic sign to indicate the course of an individual pseudotumor. Therefore, surgical excision is recommended, and should be performed as soon as is feasible.

Pathology

The basic pathology is an encapsulated blood cyst which has caused pressure necrosis of adjacent muscle and bone (Fig. 6.1). A thick fibrous tissue capsule usually surrounds a mass of gritty dark-red to brown coagulum with thick brown fluid

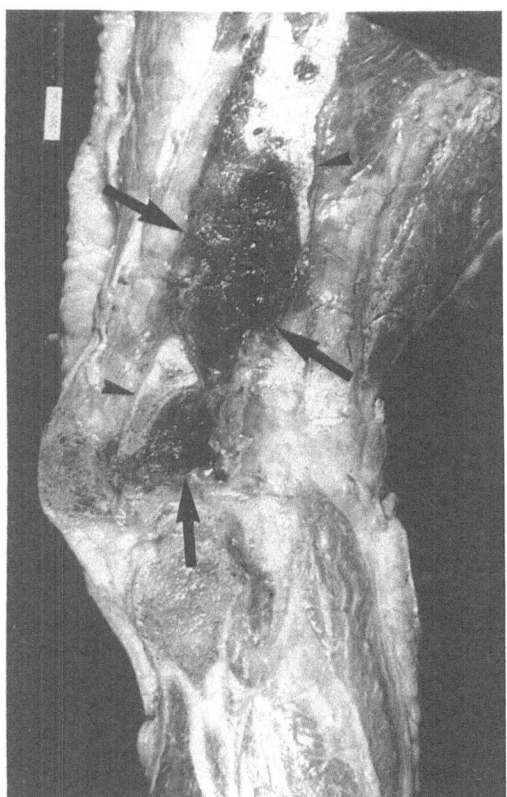

Fig. 6.1. Amputation specimen of distal femoral pseudotumor. 42-year-old with severe hemophilia A. The large multilocated blood cyst (*arrows*) has caused extensive destruction of the distal femur (*arrowheads*).

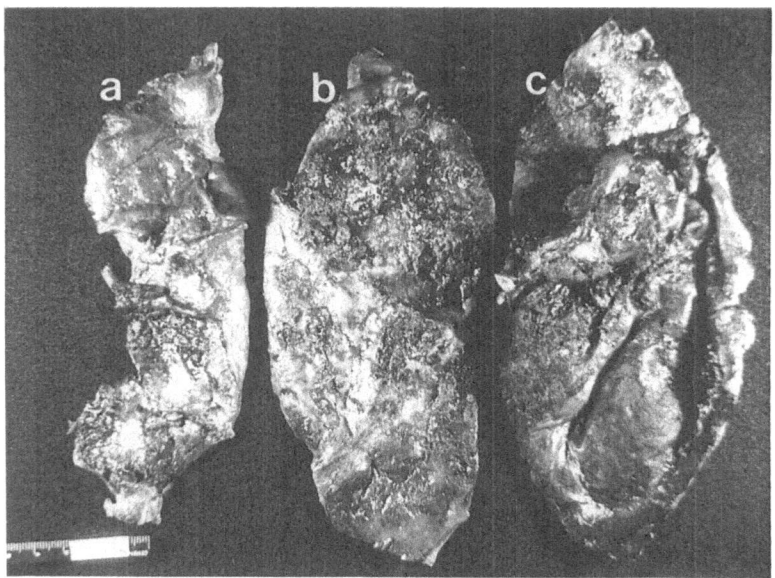

Fig. 6.2. Surgical specimen of excised femoral pseudotumor. 56-year-old with severe hemophilia A. The thick fibrous capsule is seen from the outside in *a* and *c*. *b*: the pseudotumor contents, a gritty coagulum of blood.

under low pressure (Fig. 6.2). In pseudotumors of long history the capsule is adherent to adjacent fascial attachments and may envelop neighboring neurovascular structures. The capsule overlies areas of bone necrosis and replaces the periosteum. The underlying bone is moth-eaten in appearance. In areas where periosteal stripping has occurred, large bone spicules representing new bone formation may be noted. Frequently deep daughter cysts may be seen. Many of these cysts have a thinner fibrous wall and are not very adherent to the surrounding tissues. They are frequently filled with fluid rather than coagulum and may represent an earlier stage in the evolution of a pseudotumor. Failure to recognize these daughter cysts may be the reason for the occasional recurrence noted after surgical resection.

Microscopic evaluation confirms a thick fibrous wall. de Valderrama and Matthews (1965) described a hemosiderin-filled inner layer, a dense fibrous middle layer, and a vascular outer layer. The cyst content consists of blood in various stages of degeneration and lysis. Gritty areas may be stippled with calcific debris.

de Valderrama and Matthews injected micropaque into an amputation specimen and we did a similar examination on another limb. No specific vascular abnormality was noted other than the dislocation of the main vessels and hypervascularity around the cyst. Laboratory investigation of the patients has been negative except for the coagulation deficiency, and no enzyme evaluation of cyst fluid or contents seems to be on record.

Three questions remain unanswered about the etiology of the pseudotumor. They are: (1) What is the the original site of hemorrhage in these lesions? (2) Why does the hematoma not resorb completely? and (3) What is the stimulus for the formation of the cyst wall?

Duthie et al. (1972) have stated that "hemorrhage involving bone may occur in three situations: (1) subperiosteal hemorrhage, (2) intraosseous bleeding, (3) bleeding into muscle with wide periosteal attachments." All of these have been suggested as the primary site of bleeding and pseudotumor formation. Many of the data point to the last as the site of hemorrhage of pseudotumors of the pelvis and femur. Intramuscular hemorrhage is common in hemophilia while subperiosteal hemorrhage, though reported, is rare (Moseley 1963). Soft tissue cysts without bone involvement have been demonstrated and may represent an early stage in pseudotumor development. The clinical and radiologic picture in these lesions is suggestive of extrinsic pressure necrosis of bone, and the periosteal stripping at the edge of these lesions seems to be secondary. de Valderrama and Matthews (1965), Steel et al. (1969), and Gilbert (1975) concur with this conclusion. No pathologic evidence of intraosseous bleeding has been advanced in the lesions noted above, but this etiology has been suggested in pseudotumors of the peripheral skeleton in children and will be discussed subsequently.

Diagnostic Imaging

Duthie et al. (1972) have stated that "since a haemophilic pseudotumor is clearly not a single pathologic entity, but the response of bone to a haemorrhagic process, the radiologic features will vary depending on the site and extent of the lesion."

The four characteristic radiologic features are:

1. A large soft tissue mass in proximity to bone
2. Areas of adjacent bone destruction
3. Periosteal elevation with new bone formation
4. Calcifications within the soft tissue mass

Conventional Radiography

The characteristic picture of a femoral pseudotumor as it appears on plain film radiography is shown in Figs. 6.3 and 6.4. Typical features include the large soft tissue mass, which has the same radiodensity as the surrounding muscles. However, there is obliteration of the normal fascial planes. Extensive destruction of cortical bone is noted, with several large spicules suggesting that the lesion is multilocular. In some areas the destruction is so severe that the bone seems to have lost all structural integrity. At the edges of the lesion, periosteal new bone formation may be noted. However, it is not infrequent for the soft tissue mass to extend past the area of obvious bone involvement. On review of many of these lesions one gets the impression that the necrosis of bone is extrinsic rather than intrinsic.

In another example of a proximal tibial pseudotumor (Fig. 6.5), there is an expansile metaphyseal lesion with a large extraosseous mass. The locular nature of the lesion, with calcification and ossification, should be noted.

A typical pelvic pseudotumor is seen in Fig. 6.6. The destruction of the ilium is extensive. In this area the soft tissue extent of the lesion may be difficult to evaluate, although the psoas muscle cannot be identified. Further information on the soft tissue extent may be obtained by intravenous urography (Fig. 6.7) or barium enema.

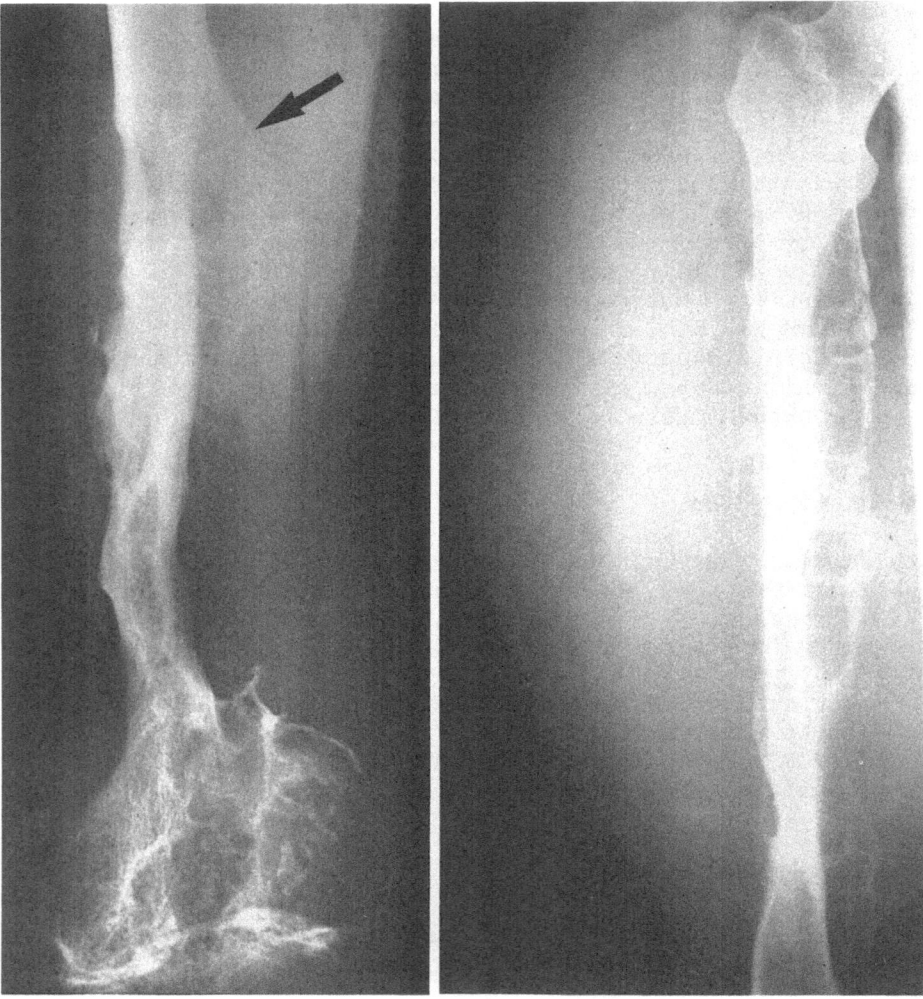

Fig. 6.3.   **Fig. 6.4.**

Fig. 6.3. Femoral pseudotumor, plain film radiography. 42-year-old with severe hemophilia A. Same patient as in Fig. 6.1. There is extensive destruction of the distal half of the femur. The bone destruction is extrinsic in nature. Periosteal new bone formation from the soft tissue mass can be seen in the cranial part of the lesion (*arrow*).

Fig. 6.4. Femoral pseudotumor, plain film radiography. 54-year-old with severe hemophilia A. The enormous extent of the soft tissue lesion, with extensive involvement of bone, can be appreciated.

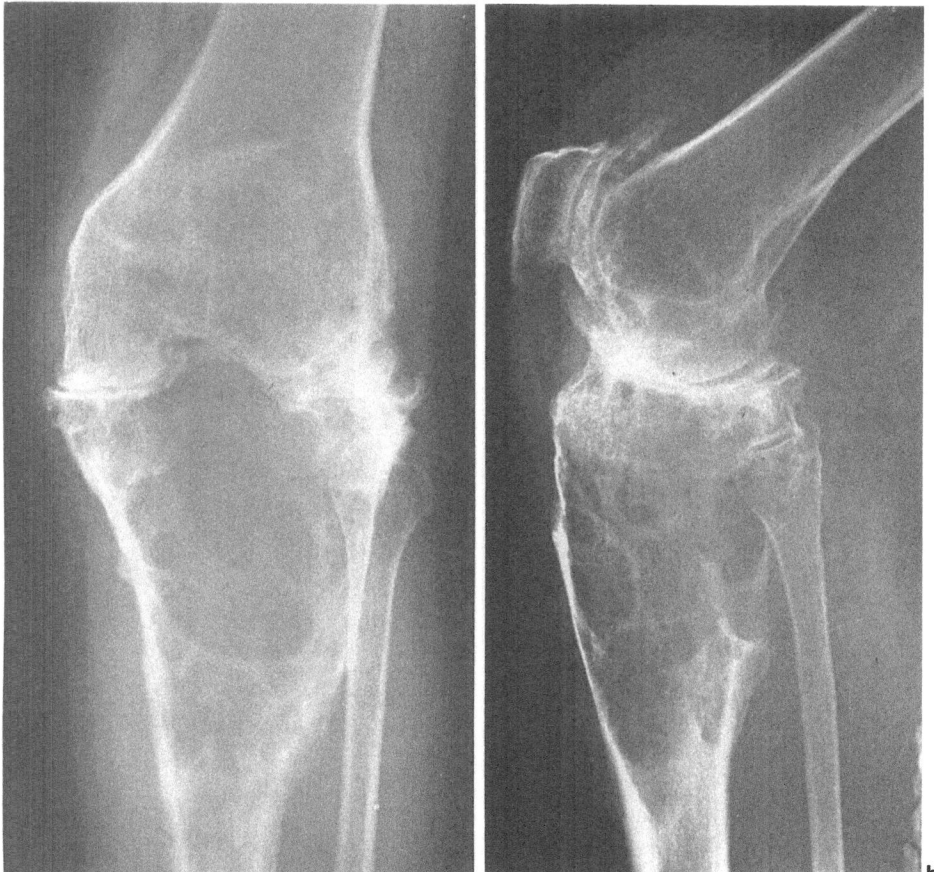

a   b

Fig. 6.5a,b. Pseudotumor of the tibia, plain film radiography. 56-year-old with severe hemophilia A. There is a large expansile metaphyseal lesion. On the lateral view the extensive soft tissue component with ossification can be seen.

Angiography may be useful in evaluating the pseudotumor. Arteriography is especially informative in assessment of pseudotumors of the extremities. Arterial puncture may be done relatively safely if good hematologic control is achieved. Factor infusion levels of 70%–100% should be achieved just before the study. If the puncture is traumatic, a second infusion 12 h later should be given. Arteriographic studies reveal displacement of the vessels (Fig. 6.8). Hyperemia may be noted at the periphery of the lesion, but there are no specific "feeding vessels" which contribute to the lesion. It should be noted that the soft tissue mass is apparently devoid of vessels. Venography has been done but has proven nonspecific except for some evidence of peripheral congestion.

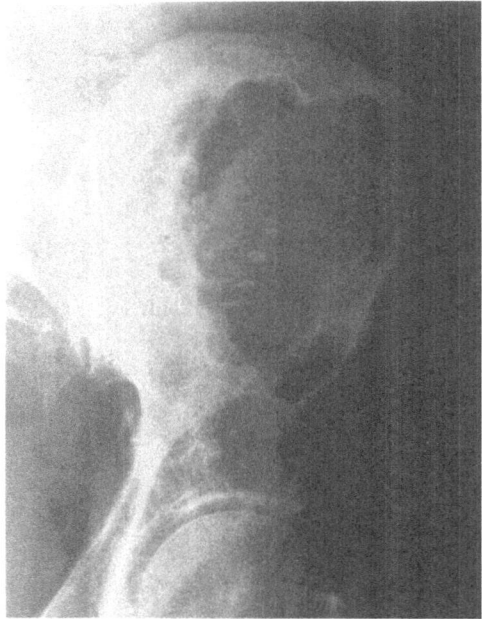

Fig. 6.6. Pseudotumor of the pelvis. 42-year-old with severe hemophilia B. Extensive destruction of the ilium. The soft tissue component is difficult to assess on the plain film.

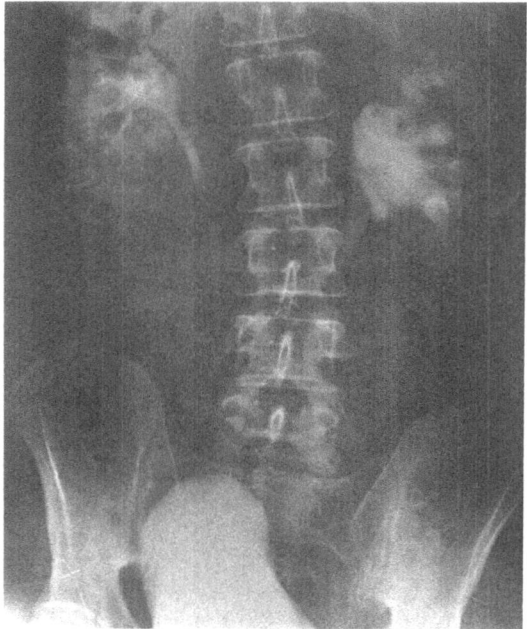

Fig. 6.7. Pseudotumor of the pelvis, intravenous urography. The large soft tissue component displaces the bladder and ureter.

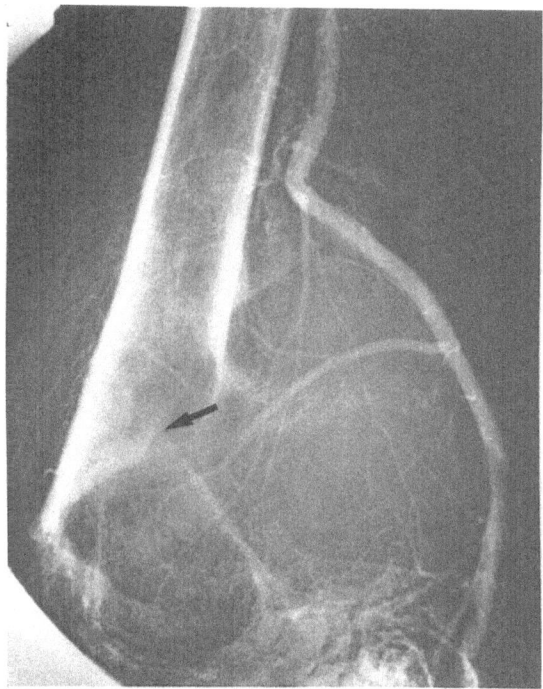

Fig. 6.8. Pseudotumor of the distal femur, arteriography, lateral view. 58-year-old with severe hemophilia A. The femoral artery and its branches are displaced by the soft tissue tumor. There is little vascularity of the tumor itself. There is a pathologic fracture through the distal femoral metaphysis (*arrow*).

Computed Tomography

Most useful in the evaluation of the hemophilic pseudotumor is computed tomography (Pettersson and Ahlberg 1982). This should be done with contrast medium injection for enhancement of the soft tissue involvement. A typical femoral lesion is seen in Fig. 6.9. The characteristic finding is a large soft tissue mass with a discrete fibrous capsule. The capsule is diagnostic of the pseudotumor and helps differentiate it from a hematoma. Equally important in the CT evaluation is the demonstration of unsuspected daughter cysts. It is common to find several of these situated in proximity to the primary lesion. It should be noted that the muscle masses surrounding the lesion are distorted and frequently thinned out. The relation of neurovascular bundles to the lesion can be seen on CT and is important in the presurgical planning. Similarly, the amount of bone destruction is easy to assess and helps in determining whether bone grafting will be required during surgery.

Computed tomographic evaluation of a pelvic pseudotumor is shown in Fig. 6.10. It is helpful to show extension into the abdominal cavity. These lesions may be extensive and can extend from the diaphragm to below the inguinal ligament.

At present we do not have any experience with magnetic resonance imaging of the hemophilic pseudotumor.

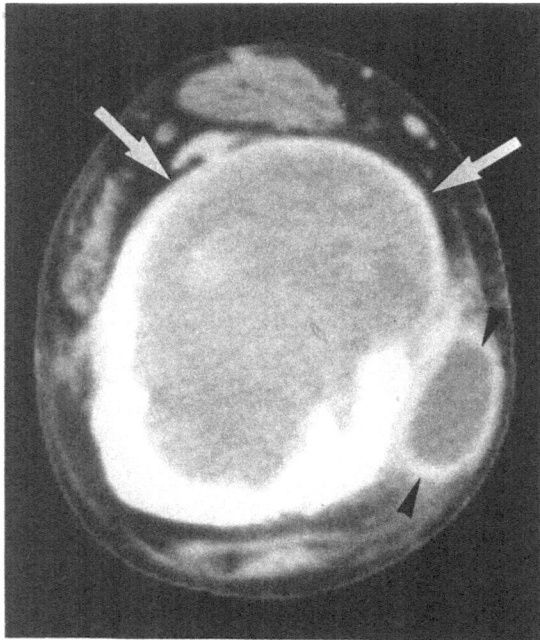

Fig. 6.9. Pseudotumor of the distal femur, CT. 40-year-old with severe hemophilia A. The large lesion involves most of the thigh. The thick fibrous capsule (*arrows*) is continuous with the expanded bone. An unsuspected daughter cyst (*arrowheads*) is situated close to the primary lesion. The muscle masses are atrophic.

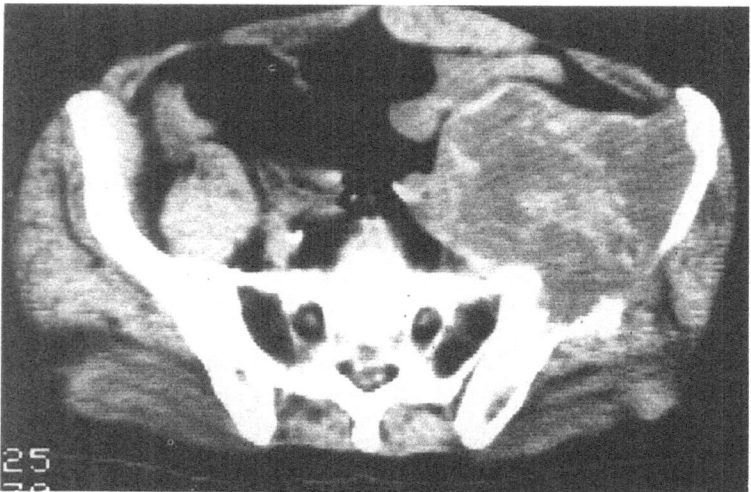

Fig. 6.10. Pelvic pseudotumor, CT. 54-year-old with severe hemophilia A. The bone destruction and the extension of the soft tissue mass into the abdominal cavity are defined. The fibrous capsule as well as calcifications within the lesion should be noted.

Protocol

For diagnosis, plain film radiography and CT are the methods of choice, and these examinations are necessary for presurgical planning. Arteriography should be performed when the pseudotumor is situated in the extremities and whenever CT reveals the possibility of vascular involvement. Retroperitoneal pseudotumors should be evaluated with intravenous urography.

The Child

Clinical Considerations

Pseudotumors in children are less common and the clinical pattern is different. A history of trauma is elicited in about one-fourth of the cases. Most often the lesions occur distal to the elbow and knee, and the large majority occur in the small bones of the hands and feet (Gilbert 1975). In contrast to the adult, where the lesions most often occur in the lower extremity, almost half of the reported lesions have been in the hand and wrist. Lesions proximal to the knee and elbow are very rare, but Hilgartner and Arnold (1975) did record a distal femoral pseudotumor in a very young child. The presentation of these tumors is also different in that progression of swelling is quite rapid. The findings are much more ominous than in adults in that the mass is warm and tender, and the overlying skin may be under tension. The lesion is usually unilocular. Pain, an unusual feature in adults, is frequently present. Another distinctive feature which may be seen is multiple involvement, with several lesions being noted either simultaneously or in rapid progression (Steel et al. 1969; Yung 1965).

The pathology of these lesions is not as well documented as it is in the adult. Surgical intervention is rarely required in that most pseudotumors in children respond to conservative modalities and surgical specimens are not available. Steel et al. (1969) reported on the pathology of a distal radial lesion and they felt that the initial site of hemorrhage was the subperiosteum. However, Gilbert (1975), after evaluating the radiographs of several other lesions, felt that the bone itself was more likely to be the site of primary bleeding.

As mentioned above, unlike the adult lesions, where surgical excision is required, many of these pseudotumors have been shown to respond to conservative care. van Creveld and Kingma (1961), MacMahon and Blackburn (1960), and Steel et al. (1969) reported peripheral pseudotumors that responded to immobilization and factor replacement. Yung (1965) recorded the eradication of bilateral tarsal pseudotumors following irradiation with a dose of 1500 rads. The femoral pseudotumor reported by Hilgartner and Arnold also responded to radiotherapy. Brant and Jordan (1972) had previously reported on the efficacy of radiotherapy in adult pseudotumors, but complete eradication of the lesion was not demonstrated and personal follow-up on several of these patients showed subsequent progression with the need for surgical removal. Because of the above experiences it is our suggestion that pseudotumors in the immature skeleton be treated with immobilization and factor replacement. If there is not a good response, local irradiation should be considered.

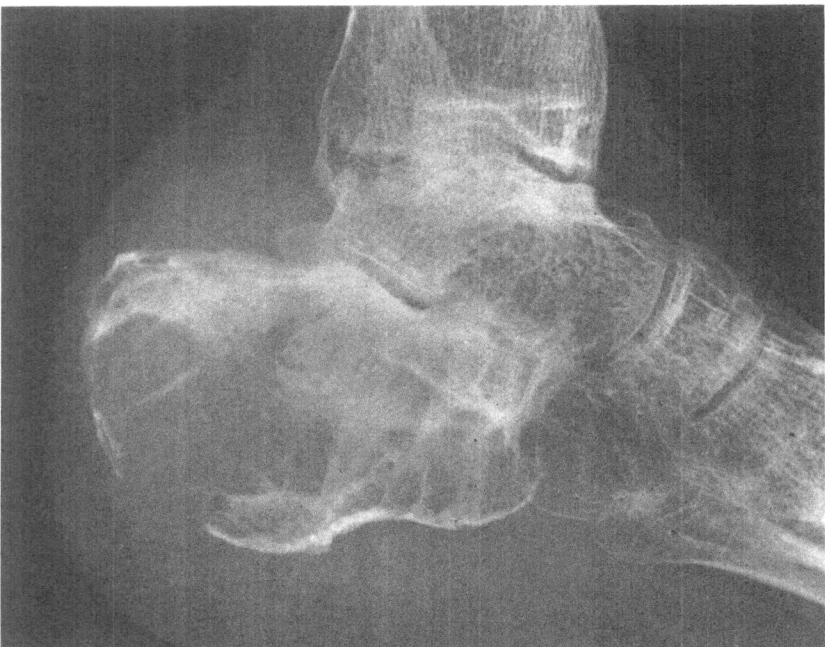

Fig. 6.11. Pseudotumor of the calcaneus, plain film radiography. 14-year-old with severe hemophilia A. There is an expansile lesion with thinning and breakthrough of the cortex and destruction of the trabecular pattern. The soft tissue component is less prominent than in adult lesions.

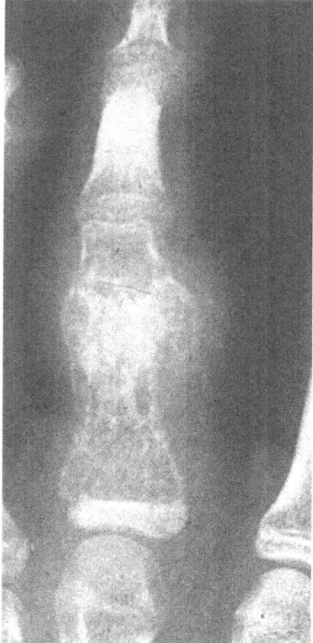

Fig. 6.12. Pseudotumor of the third finger. 13-year-old with hemophilia A. There is an expansile lesion of the proximal phalanx with thinning of the cortex. No significant soft tissue mass is evident.

Diagnostic Imaging

The radiologic picture differs from that in the adult as there is no large soft tissue component and the lesion appears to be expansile from within the bone. Internal destruction of the normal trabecular pattern is noted, with aneurysmal expansion of the cortex. The cortex may be fractured or destroyed and at times the picture is compatible with infection or malignancy. A coarse trabecular pattern can be seen within the lesion. In the bones of the hands and feet there is no evidence of new bone formation. Periosteal new bone formation with a large soft tissue component was a feature of the distal radial pseudotumor reported by Steel et al. (1969) and the femoral pseudotumor reported by Hilgartner and Arnold (1975). The characteristics described above are shown in Figs. 6.11 and 6.12.

Following treatment it is impressive to see how much reconstitution of normal bone is possible. However, some persistent deformity is usually noted (Fig. 6.13).

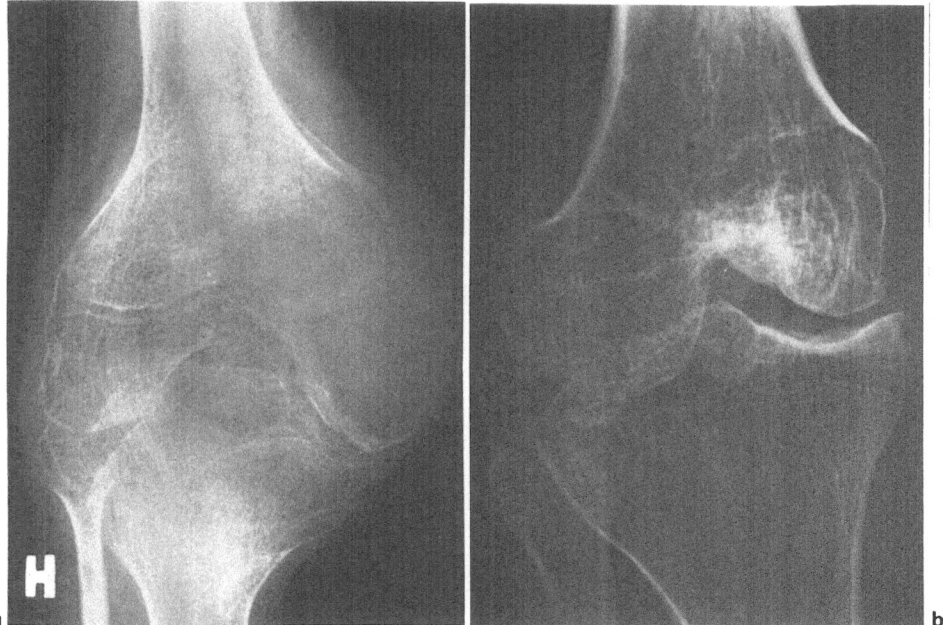

a   b

Fig. 6.13a,b. Pseudotumor of the distal femur in a child, healed following factor replacement therapy. Hemophilia A. **a** At 10 years of age there is a large expansile lesion within the medial femoral condyle, destroying the trabecular pattern and the cortex. The growth plate is involved. *b* 4 years later the lesion has healed after factor replacement therapy, but the growth is disturbed.

References

Ahlberg Å (1975) On the natural history of hemophilic pseudotumor. J Bone Joint Surg [Am] 57: 1133–1136
Brant EE, Jordan MH (1972) Radiologic aspects of hemophilic pseudotumors in bone. AJR 115: 525–539

de Valderrama JAF, Matthews JM (1965) The haemophilic pseudotumour or haemophilic subperiosteal haematoma. J Bone Joint Surg [Br] 47: 256–265

Duthie RB, Matthews JM, Rizza CR, Steel WM (1972) The management of musculo-skeletal problems in the haemophilias. Blackwell Scientific, Oxford

Gilbert MS (1975) Haemophilic pseudotumor. In: Brinkhous KM, Hemker HC (eds) Handbook of haemophilia. Excerpta Medica, Amsterdam

Gunning AJ (1966) The surgery of haemophilic cysts. In: Biggs R, MacFarlane RG (eds) Treatment of haemophilia and other coagulation disorders. Blackwell Scientific, Oxford

Hilgartner MW, Arnold WD (1975) Hemophiliac pseudotumor treated with replacement and radiation therapy. J Bone Joint Surg [Am] 57: 1145–1148

MacMahon JS, Blackburn CRB (1960) Haemophilic pseudotumor; a report of a case treated conservatively. Aust NZ J Surg, 29: 129–131

Martinson A (1976) Hemophilic pseudotumors. In: Boone DC (ed) Comprehensive management of hemophilia. F.A. Davis, Philadelphia

Moseley JE (1963) Bone changes in hematologic disorders. Grune and Stratton, New York London

Pettersson H, Ahlberg Å (1982) Computed tomography in hemophilic pseudotumor. Acta Radiol (Diagn) 23: 453–457

Starker L (1918) Knochenusur durch ein hämophiles subperiostales Hämatoma. Mitt Grenzgeb Med Chir 31: 381–385

Steel WM, Duthie RB, O'Connor BT (1969) Haemophilic cysts. Report of five cases. J Bone Joint Surg [Br] 51: 614–626

van Creveld S, Kingma MJ (1961) Subperiosteal hemorrhage in haemophilia A and B. Acta Paediatr Scand 50: 291–296

Yung Fu Chen (1965) Bilateral hemophilic pseudotumors of the calcaneus and cuboid treated by irradiation: Case report. J Bone Joint Surg [Am] 47: 517–521

Chapter 7

Fractures

The literature on the management of fracture problems in hemophilia is at times contradictory, but it is our clinical impression and the impression of several authors that fractures are not uncommon, that they rarely cause significant bleeding problems, and that union occurs in a normal manner. The principles of good fracture management should be followed and only modified in that initial hemostasis must be achieved and maintained by factor replacement. Conservative care is preferable, but open reduction is indicated where the fracture necessitates this for achievement and maintenance of reduction. Good fracture care demands that restrictive bandages be avoided if possible in the face of significant swelling and that the neurovascular status be closely monitored. Any analysis of the literature must take into account that many of the reports discuss fractures that occurred before the availability of adequate factor replacement.

Incidence

Feil et al., (1974) stated that fractures in hemophilia are rare. Flatmark in 1964 and Ahlberg and Nilsson in 1967 reported on 18 and 20 patients respectively. Boardman and English (1980) reported on 22 patients with fractures and dislocations during a 9-year period which ended in 1978. These fractures occurred in a population of 580 patients. At the Mount Sinai Hospital where we follow over 400 hemophiliacs, 44 have sustained a fracture during their lifetime. Thus the incidence of fractures in hemophilia is considerable.

Site of Fracture and Severity of Trauma

An inordinate number of fractures occur about the hip and knee if the young age of the population is taken into account (Ahlberg and Nilsson 1967; Boardman and English 1980; Feil et al. 1974; Flatmark 1964; Ikkala 1960; Jordan 1958). This is especially true in those series which appeared before adequate treatment became available. Broadman and English (1980) also noted that an increased number of fractures occurred in those patients with severe hemophilia, often following minor trauma (Fig. 7.1). They recorded three transcervical fractures of the femur from minor falls to the side. We have followed a patient who developed a stress fracture with minimal walking activity. Many of the fractures occurred in patients with radiologic changes of hemophilic arthropathy (Fig. 7.2). Similarly, fractures about the knee, especially in the supracondylar area, occurred from a moderate flexion force or a minor fall (Fig. 7.3). Fractures about the ankle, a common site in the normal population, were not common. The sites of 52 fractures in patients followed at the Mount Sinai Hospital are shown in Table 7.1.

Table 7.1. Fractures, Mt. Sinai Hospital

Site	No.
Femur: hip	9
shaft	8
supracondylar	11
Tibia/fibula	10
Radius/ulna	10
Humerus	1
Clavicle	2
Ribs	1
	52 (44 patients)

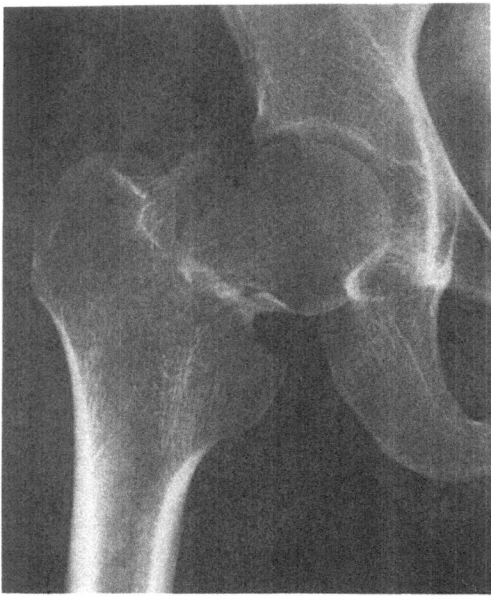

Fig. 7.1. Fracture of the femoral neck. 19-year-old with severe hemophilia A. The fracture was sustained with minimal trauma. The diagnosis was not made until 10 days later because the patient thought he had a hemarthrosis of the hip.

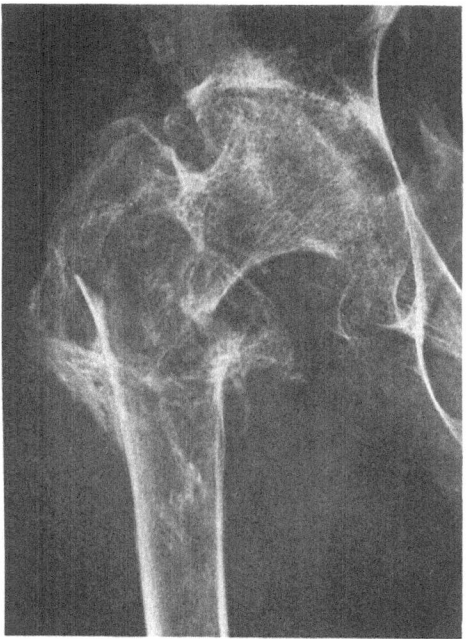

Fig. 7.2. Intertrochanteric fracture. 24-year-old with severe hemophilia A. The radiograph demonstrates the arthropathy and osteoporosis frequently associated with fractures in hemophiliacs.

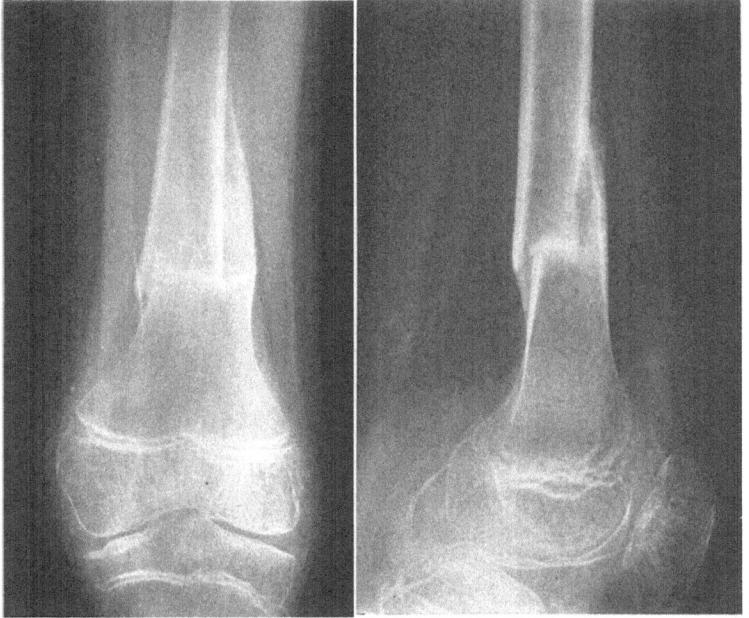

Fig. 7.3a,b. Fracture of the distal femur. 14-year-old with severe hemophilia A. This healing fracture was sustained when the patient tripped and forced his knee into flexion.

Many of the fractures reported in the literature and in our series were not diagnosed immediately following the trauma. Because the trauma was minimal and the patient thought he was experiencing a hemarthrosis, radiographs were not obtained. Therefore it is our recommendation that radiographic examination be considered in most trauma to the extremities.

Most authors have pointed out that the unusual pattern of fractures is due to three factors:

1. Limitation of the joint motion
2. Osteoporosis
3. Poor muscle function, especially at the quadriceps

There is little question that these changes are the result of recurrent hemarthroses, especially at the knee. Weakness of the quadriceps, with secondary buckling, may be a consequence of the arthropathy or of a femoral neuropathy associated with iliacus hemorrhage.

The pattern of fractures just described is becoming less common as patients are treating hemarthroses early and are beginning to participate in sports. Many of the fractures seen in the past 5 years have occurred about the wrist and ankle and are the result of bona fide trauma. In addition, a number of serious fractures have been associated with motor vehicle accidents.

Bleeding

Bleeding has not proven to be a significant problem in fracture treatment in the hemophiliac patient. As recently as 1959, nevertheless, Coventry et al. did report severe life-threatening bleeding following a fracture of the femur. Ahlberg and Nilsson (1967) attributed complications to increased bleeding in over half their reported fractures. However, they seemed to be very critical of their results and in general their patients did quite well. Most other authors comment on the ease with which bleeding is controlled. If the trauma was not severe, excellent hemostasis was achieved in most cases, with factor being required for less than 1 week. With unstable or open fractures or following major trauma, such as from a motor vehicle accident, increased bleeding has been noted but can be controlled if sufficient factor levels are achieved.

Union

All authors agree that fractures in hemophilia unite in average time. Following reports of delayed union with anticoagulant therapy, there was concern that fracture healing in hemophilia might be delayed, but Flatmark (1964) showed that union occurred in normal time. Jordan (1958) had suggested that union may even be accelerated, but there is little evidence to support this. Malunions and nonunions have been reported in the past, but these were mainly due to inadequate fracture care and not to the hemorragic diathesis (Fig. 7.4).

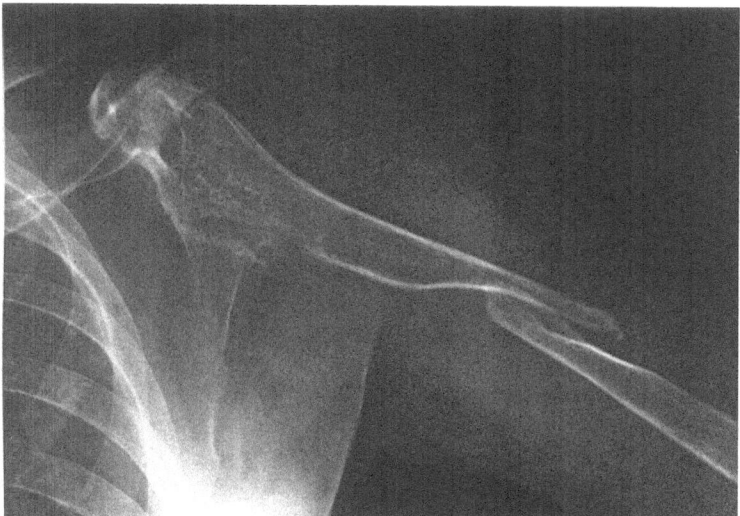

Fig. 7.4. Pseudarthrosis of the humerus. 64-year-old with severe hemophilia A. This established nonunion occurred 20 years earlier. The immobilization was inadequate because of the fear of hemorrhagic complications.

Feil et al. (1974) and Kemp and Matthews (1968) commented upon the paucity of callus in many of these patients and felt that healing in hemophilia was largely endosteal. Boardman and English (1980) demonstrated normal callus formation in many of their fractures. We believe that the lack of exuberant callus in the earlier cases was the result of fractures with minimal periosteal stripping. There is no reason to suspect that fractures heal in a different manner in hemophilia than they do in the normal population.

Pseudotumor Formation

Harrison in 1964 reported on the development of a pseudotumor following fracture of the femur. This occurred at a time when adequate hematologic control was not available. Since pseudotumors can evolve following bleeding into large muscle masses, it is not at all surprising that a pseudotumor could develop following a fracture of the femur. In addition, there is some speculation that pseudotumors do develop from subperiosteal hemorrhage and we know that this does occur following this type of fracture. There are other reports of fractures associated with pseudotumors, but upon analysis most of these appear to be fractures which occurred through a bone compromised by a preexisting pseudotumor (Fig. 6.8). However, the radiologist must bear in mind that pseudotumors may develop following fractures in hemophilia, and therefore radiologic follow-up of all fractures is required (Fig. 7.5). The fractures should be followed until solid union has occurred. Evidence of persistent soft tissue swelling, calcification, or persistent periosteal elevation should be evaluated by computed tomography.

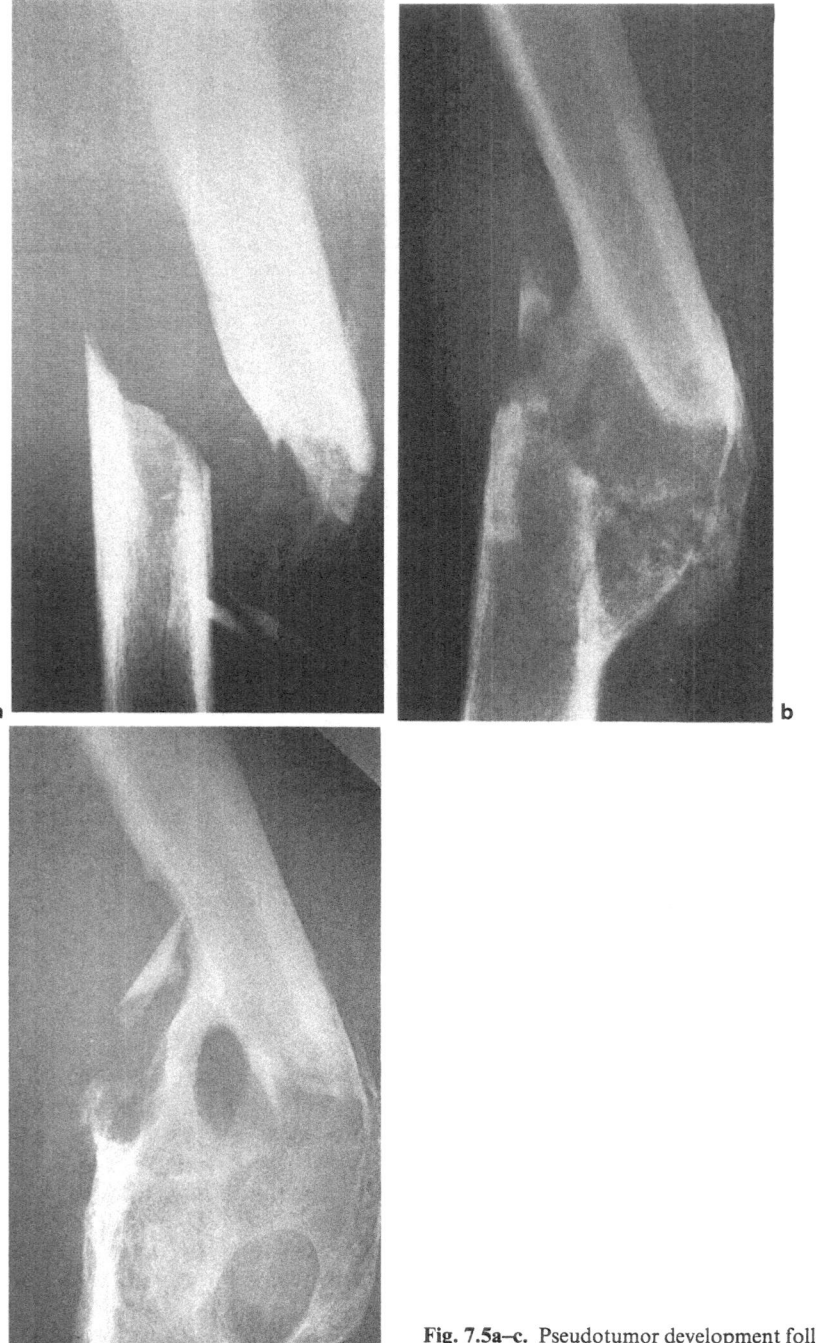

Fig. 7.5a–c. Pseudotumor development following fracture of the femur. **a** Age 32, displaced fracture of the femur. **b** Age 39, healed, with beginning pseudotumor formation. **c** Age 46, pseudotumor formation at the fracture site and within the distal fragment.

References

Ahlberg Å, Nilsson IM (1967) Fractures in hemophiliacs with special reference to complications and treatment. Acta Chir Scand 133: 293–302

Boardman KP, English P (1980) Fractures and dislocations in hemophilia. Clin Orthop 148: 221–232

Coventry MB, Owen CA, Murphy TR, Miles SD (1959) Survival of patient with hemophilia and fracture of femur. J Bone Joint Surg [Am] 41: 1392–1398

Feil E, Bentley G, Rizza CR (1974) Fracture management in patients with haemophilia. J Bone Joint Surg [Br] 56: 643–649

Flatmark AL (1964) Fracture union in the presence of delayed blood coagulation. Acta Chir Scand (Suppl) 344

Harrison JF (1964) Haemophilic pseudotumor after fracture femur. Br Med J I: 544

Ikkala E (1960) Haemophilia. Scand J Clin Lab Invest 12 (Suppl): 46

Jordan HH (1958) Hemophilic Arthropathies. Charles Thomas, Springfield, Ill

Kemp HS, Matthews JM (1968) The management of fractures in haemophilia and Christmas disease. J Bone Joint Surg [Br] 50: 351–381

Chapter 8
The Central Nervous System

Intracranial Hemorrhage

Bleeding into the cranial cavity has always been a serious threat to the hemophilic patient and the main cause of death in this patient group (Aledort 1976; Bacher 1980; Larsson and Wiechel 1983). Before the modern era of treatment, the mortality after intracranial bleeding was estimated at 70% (Silverstein 1960; van Trotzenburg 1975). Modern treatment has changed these figures, but still the incidence in several publications has been high and in a recent report on deaths in Swedish hemophiliacs from 1957 to 1980, 37 of 118 deaths were caused by intracranial hemorrhage (Larsson and Wiechel 1983). This is in accordance with Eyster et al. (1978) and Federici (1982), who estimated the mortality in adults after intracranial hemorrhage to be 30%–40%. In children it seems to be lower (Pettersson et al. 1984). Of adult survivors, about 50% are left with neurologic sequelae (Eyster et al. 1978), while the potential for clinical recovery is greater in young patients (Bruce 1978; Pettersson et al. 1984; Seeler and Imana 1973; Silverstein 1960).

Clinical Aspects

The age at which intracranial bleeding occurs varies, but it is most frequent in children and youngsters (Eyster et al. 1978). A few cases have been reported in which intracranial hemorrhage in the newborn period was the first sign of hemophilia, and indeed the reason for hematologic workup and diagnosis (Pettersson et al. 1984; Volpe et al. 1976).

In half of the cases there was no known injury, and in those with known trauma there was often a delay between the trauma and the occurrence of symptoms, varying between 1 day and several weeks (Eyster et al. 1978). This delay is well known in neurosurgical practice when dealing with subdural hematomas in other patients, but in hemophiliacs it is also seen in bleeding into the other compartments of the cranial cavity. The delay in the onset of symptoms is typical for this patient group as a minute cerebral contusion after mild injury may continue to enlarge gradually, owing to the coagulation defect.

Patients with subarachnoid hemorrhage usually present with headache and stiff neck, or with other signs of meningeal irritation. Patients with subdural intracranial bleeding, with or without known trauma and with or without a delay between the trauma and the symptoms, may also present with headache, nausea and vomiting, and signs of meningeal irritation, which may progress to coma. Seizures, irritability or confusion, blurred vision, or any other signs of intracranial damage may be presenting symptoms (Eyster et al. 1978), and any persistent unexplained headache in a hemophiliac must be suspected to indicate intracranial hemorrhage (Curless and Corrigan 1976; Forster 1981; Kerr 1964; van Trotzenburg 1975; Visconti and Hilgartner 1980).

Bleeding is equally common in the subdural, subarachnoid, and intracerebral compartments, while extradural hemorrhage is rare (Eyster et al. 1978; Federici et al. 1982; Larsson and Wiechel 1983). The bleeding usually occurs into the supratentorial space, and posterior fossa hematomas are seldom seen (Raggio et al. 1978; Moody and Mullan 1968).

Recurrence of the bleeding is relatively common, in accordance with the general tendency in hemophiliacs to rebleed in an area of previous hemorrhage (Silverstein 1960). In Eyster's material (1978) such recurrent bleeding was reported in 20% of the cases.

Prompt diagnosis and treatment is of utmost importance, and today CT of the skull should be performed whenever suspicion of intracranial hemorrhage is raised in a hemophilic patient.

Diagnostic Imaging

Prior to the era of CT, the modalities available for confirmation or exclusion of intracranial bleeding were brain scintimetry, electroencephalography, cerebral angiography, and lumbar puncture. Of these, electroencephalography and brain scan could be performed without any risk to the patient and without correction of the hemostatic defect.

Cerebral Angiography

With cerebral angiography, changes in the position and structure of the vessels may reveal the intracranial hemorrhage. *Subdural hematoma* has a characteristic appearance, as the interposition of blood between the surface of the brain and the inner table of the scalp leaves an area totally void of vessels. Also, the midline vessels such as the pericallosal artery and the internal cerebral vein will be dislocated towards the opposite side (Fig. 8.1). The angiographic changes in *extradural hematomas* are similar to those of subdural bleeding, although in the extradural hematoma the meningeal arteries are dislocated together with the cerebral arteries (Cronqvist and Köhler 1963). *Intracerebral hematomas* may give rise to angiographic changes illustrative of the expansile character of the lesion. Thus the vessels will be dislocated in a manner that depends on the localization of the lesion (Greitz and Lindgren 1971). Intracerebral hemorrhage as well as *subarachnoid bleeding* may cause spasm of the vessels running into or near the lesion. Such spasm is most often found in the carotid siphon and in the main brain branches of the anterior and middle cerebral arteries.

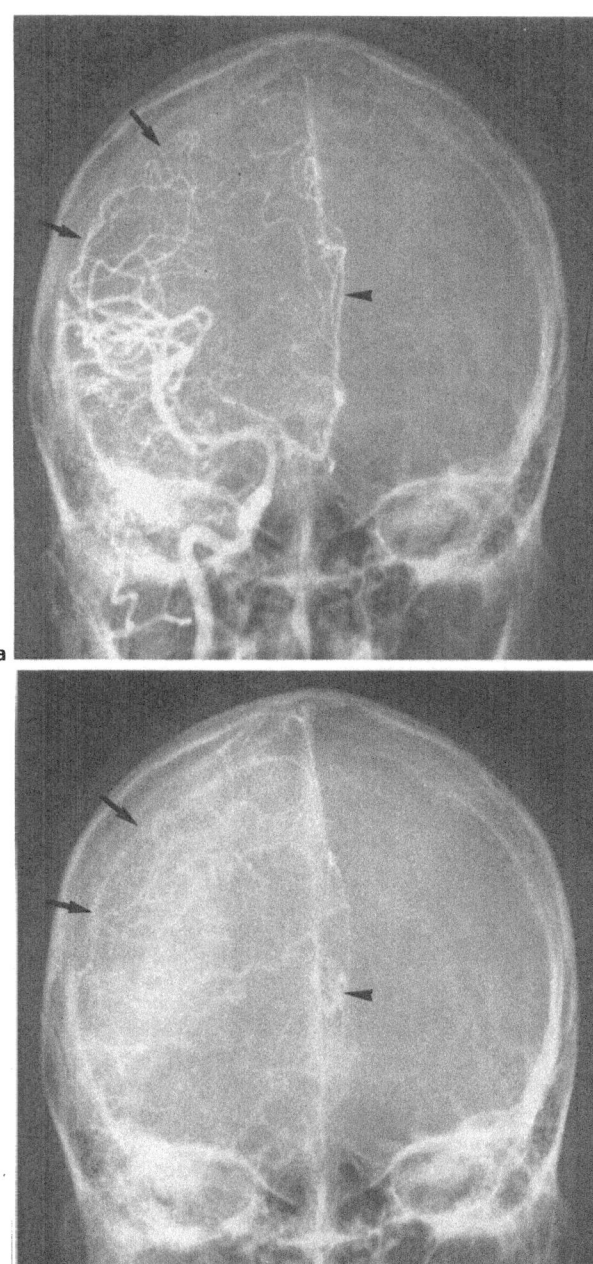

Fig. 8.1a,b. Subdural hematoma, cerebral angiography. 16-year-old with severe hemophilia A. **a** arterial and **b** venous phase. The hematoma is interposed between the surface of the brain and the inner table of the skull, leaving an area void of vessels (*arrows*). The anterior cerebral artery, the pericallosal artery (*arrowhead*), and the central vein (*arrowhead*) are dislocated past the midline.

The angiographic examination, of course, must be performed under cover of factor replacement. With proper factor levels (70%–100%), the complication rate should be equal to that for angiography in other patient groups. Only one fatal postangiographic complication in a hemophiliac is on record (Simpson and Robson 1960). That patient had a percutaneous carotid approach and died of massive bleeding. He had received fresh-frozen plasma before the examination, but the factor VIII level after infusion was only 10%.

Computed Tomography

Today, computed tomography has replaced the above diagnostic modalities. It is a noninvasive examination, performed with ease for the patient and giving all the necessary information on the presence, location, and extent of intracranial bleeding. The great value of CT in the diagnostic workup of intracranial hemorrhage in hemophilia has been reported by several authors (Federici et al. 1982; Forster 1981; Gore et al. 1981; Kinney et al. 1977; Matsuda et al. 1977; Newland et al. 1979; Yoshida et al. 1979; Zouaoui et al. 1980).

The attenuation value of the brain tissue is about 30–40 HU, while fresh clotted blood has attenuation values varying between 50 and 70 HU, mainly owing to the protein fractions of hemoglobin (Ambrose 1973; New et al. 1974). With hemolysis the attenuation value decreases (Ambrose 1974; Cronqvist et al. 1975; Levander et al. 1975) and thus it is important to know the time between trauma and examination. The edema which may surround a hematoma is represented by an area of decreased attenuation.

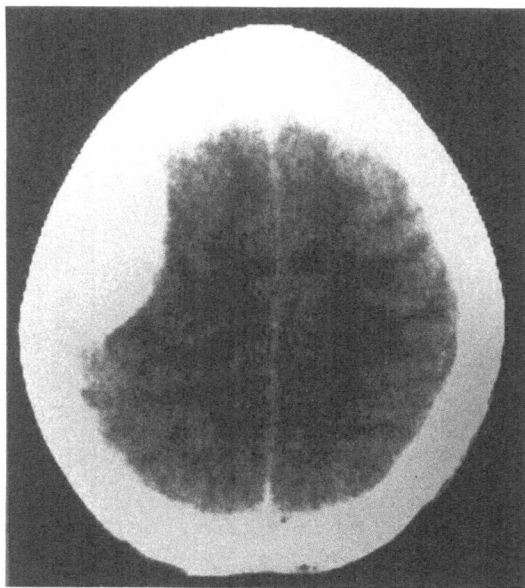

Fig. 8.2. Epidural hematoma, computed tomography. 14-year-old with severe hemophilia A. The blood collection forms a biconvex area of increased density between the brain and the skull.

Classically, acute *epidural hematoma* presents as a biconvex area of increased density (Fig. 8.2), while acute *subdural hematoma* is convex externally and concave internally (Fig. 8.3a). With hemolysis of the blood, the attenuation value diminishes, and in a patient with normal hemostasis the blood in the hematoma is isodense with the brain tissue between 1 and 3 weeks following the trauma (Fig. 8.3b). After this, the attenuation value of the extracerebral hematoma is lower than the brain but slightly higher than the cerebrospinal fluid (CSF) (Dolinskas et al. 1977), and remains so for a long time. On the other hand, the hematoma

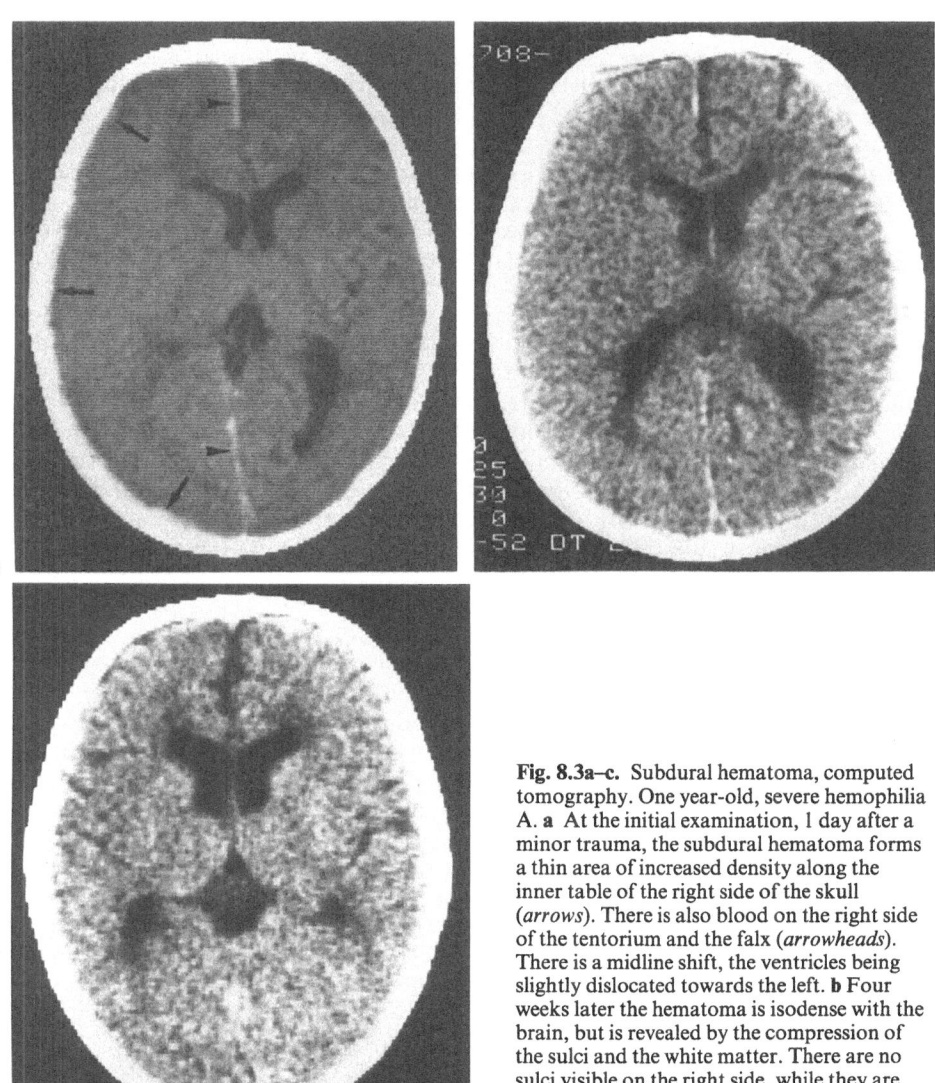

Fig. 8.3a–c. Subdural hematoma, computed tomography. One year-old, severe hemophilia A. **a** At the initial examination, 1 day after a minor trauma, the subdural hematoma forms a thin area of increased density along the inner table of the right side of the skull (*arrows*). There is also blood on the right side of the tentorium and the falx (*arrowheads*). There is a midline shift, the ventricles being slightly dislocated towards the left. **b** Four weeks later the hematoma is isodense with the brain, but is revealed by the compression of the sulci and the white matter. There are no sulci visible on the right side, while they are normal on the left side. **c** Normal CT of the brain 3 months after the injury.

may totally resolve and the CT appearance return to normal (Fig. 8.3c). In hemophiliacs the time schedule for this change in attenuation values may be disturbed because of refilling of the hematoma with fresh blood. Thus, the isodense period may be longer, making diagnosis more difficult (Fig. 8.3b). However, there are several secondary signs that may reveal the hematoma, such as displacement of the ventricles and compression of the sulci and the white matter (Fig. 8.3b). If there is any doubt about the CT diagnosis the examination should be repeated after injection of intravenous contrast medium, as the contrast medium will enhance the inner membrane of the hematoma, giving a clear separation of the hematoma and brain tissue (Omar and Binet 1978).

Intracerebral hematomas in the acute stage appear as lesions with increased density, often surrounded by a rim of lower attenuation caused by edema (Fig. 8.4a,b). Again, the density of these hematomas will diminish with time, and in the end stage there may be a circumscribed fluid collection with an attenuation value slightly above that of CSF (Fig. 8.4c,d). Large hematomas in the end stage are usually surrounded by a thin area of gliosis. Small hematomas may heal with a scar that may not be possible to see on the CT examination, but focal atrophy or ventricular enlargement may reveal the sequelae of bleeding.

Subarachnoid hemorrhage may be revealed by attenuation values of cisterns and sulci that are isodense or hyperdense compared with the brain tissue (de Villasante and Taveras 1976).

The CT appearance of *cerebral contusion* overlaps with intracerebral hematoma on the one hand and with cerebral edema on the other. It is usually seen as a mottled area of increased density, mixed with areas of edema. If the lesion is large it will cause a mass effect on surrounding structures.

Computed tomography is of importance not only for the detection of intracranial bleeding but also for the follow-up of hemophiliacs who have sustained trauma. It is also of great importance in the period immediately after surgical intervention, as there is a considerable risk of early recurrence, especially in patients in whom the coagulation state is difficult to control (Fig. 8.5). As recurrence of the hemorrhage may develop slowly, repeat CT examination should be performed at the slightest change in the clinical status.

Later *sequelae*, such as hygromas, fluid-filled cysts, or hydrocephalus, may develop, giving neurologic disturbances (Federici et al. 1982; Matsuda et al. 1977; McCarthy and Coble 1973); again CT can be used to demonstrate the lesion.

The *long-term sequelae* of intracranial bleeding have hitherto not been known, although in most reports about half of the survivors have been left with neurologic disturbances (Eyster et al. 1978). Recently we reviewed nine hemophiliac children who had sustained an intracranial hemorrhage. They had follow-up evaluation both clinically and with CT 4–17 (mean 8.6) years after the hemorrhage. The structural damage as seen on CT was in most cases more pronounced than was expected clinically. Posthemorrhagic or postsurgical cerebral malacia with porencephalic cysts, enlarged ventricles, and an enlarged subarachnoid space was seen in almost all patients, and such damage was present in several patients who had no or minimal clinical sequelae (Fig. 8.4c,d). The cerebral malacia was more pronounced than would be expected, possibly being caused by disturbed healing due to the clotting defect (Pettersson et al. 1984).

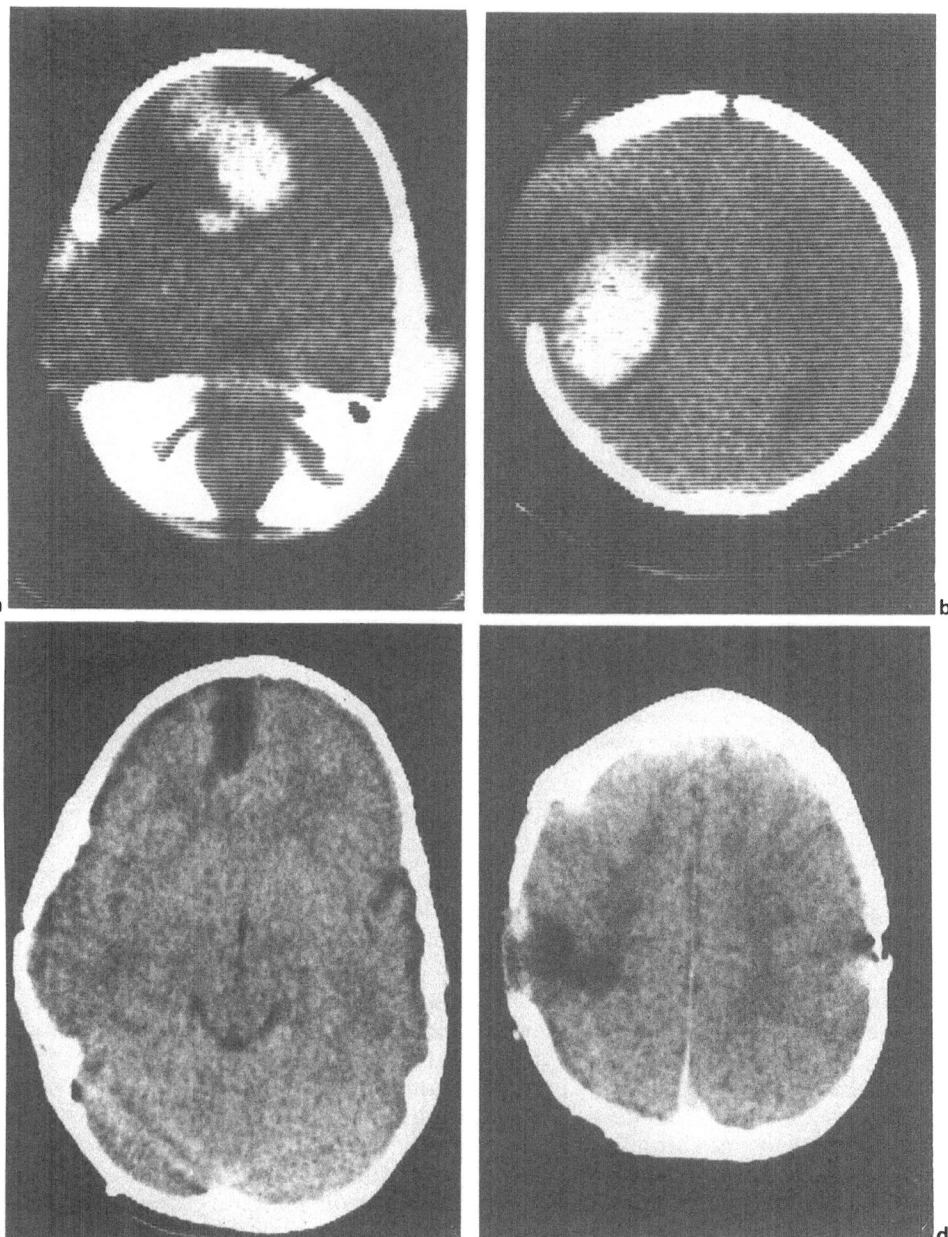

Fig. 8.4. Intracerebral hematomas, computed tomography. **a,b** 6-month-old with severe hemophilia A. A large defect is present in the skull after an exploratory craniotomy performed 1 day before the CT examination. There is a large right frontal hematoma with extension over the midline into the left hemisphere (**a**), and a large right parietal hematoma (**b**). Around the frontal hematoma there is pronounced edema (*arrows*). The edema around the parietal hematoma is smaller. **c,d** Follow-up examination 3 years later, when the patient was clinically totally normal. A porencephalic cavity is seen in the right frontal and the right parietal hemispheres. (From Pettersson et al. 1984, with permission.)

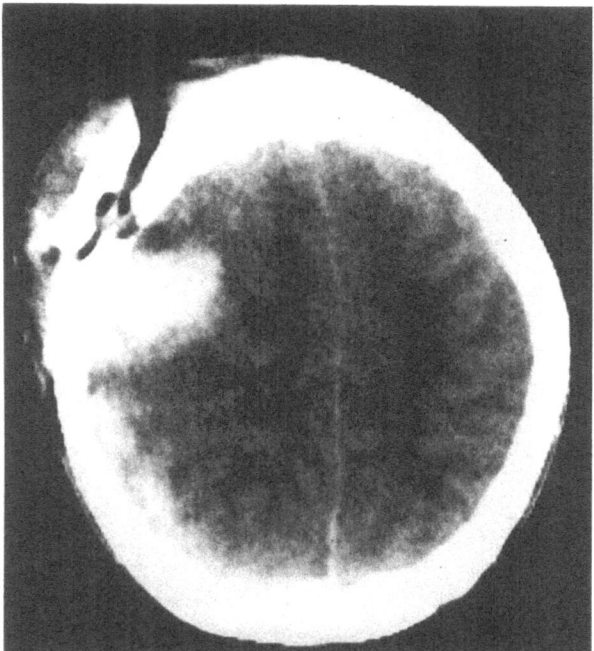

Fig. 8.5. Recurrent hemorrhage after surgical intervention. 14-year-old with severe hemophilia A. The patient had a subdural hematoma evacuated 3 days before this CT examination. His clinical state deteriorated, and a repeat CT examination revealed intracranial and subdural bleeding.

Diagnostic Protocol for Head Trauma or Suspected Intracranial Hemorrhage

Computed tomography is a rapid and safe examination, making possible prompt and adequate surgical intervention when needed. In patients in whom observation is elected, the development of intracerebral bleeding will be detected at repeat CT examination, again leading to prompt therapy. In accordance with Gore et al. (1981) we therefore recommend the following approach to the diagnostic workup of hemophiliacs with head trauma or suspected intracranial bleeding.

Adequate factor replacement should be instituted immediately in all such patients. If the trauma is small and there are no neurologic disturbances, only clinical observation is needed. If there are neurologic changes or if the trauma is more severe, CT should be performed. If the CT is negative, the patient should be observed clinically, with replacement therapy for at least a week to prevent delayed bleeding. If CT at that time is still normal, the patient may be discharged. If the CT demonstrates intracranial hemorrhage, and if after neurosurgical consultation further observation is elected, repeat CT examination at appropriate intervals must be performed. If surgery is performed, CT will be of value in the postoperative period as described above.

Intraspinal Hemorrhage

Bleeding into the spinal canal is rare (Cromwell et al. 1977; Harvie et al. 1977; Keely et al. 1972; Abad Rico et al. 1979; Schiller et al. 1948; Stanley and McComb 1983; Sumner 1962). Since the first report by Tellegen (1850), only about 20 cases are on record. Among the 580 patients with hemophilia in Sweden in 1984, there are two who have sustained intraspinal bleeding, both with neurologic sequelae (Nilsson and Blombäck, personal communication).

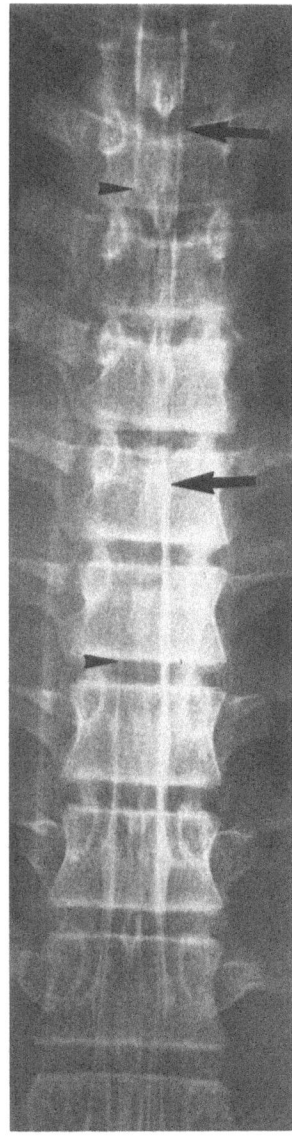

Fig. 8.6. Intraspinal hemorrhage, conventional myelography. There is a large extradural hematoma at the left side extending over several vertebral levels and displacing the dural sac to the right (*arrows*). The cord and sac are pressed towards the right wall of the spinal canal, so that no contrast medium passes in this side of the subarachnoid space over four vertebral levels of the sac (*arrowheads*).

A known injury has been reported in less than one-third of the cases (Harvie et al. 1977; van Trotzenburg 1975). When the hemorrhage occurs, the symptoms are rapidly progressive, with violent radicular pain from either the neck or the back. The pain may subside for a short while, but soon returns with rapid loss of neurologic function (Keely et al. 1972; van Trotzenburg 1975). Very rarely the course may be chronic, the symptoms being the same as with other lesions that compress the spinal cord, such as tumor, abscess, or intervertebral disc prolapse (Keely et al. 1972).

The outcome of intraspinal hemorrhage is variable, but in general the prognosis is bad (Harvie et al. 1977). Of the survivors, most are left with paraplegia or tetraparesis (Harvie et al. 1977; Mamoli et al. 1976; Schiller et al. 1948), although excellent recovery has been reported in some cases (Cromwell et al. 1977; Stanley and McComb 1983).

If bleeding into the spinal canal is suspected, factor replacement should be instituted immediately, and under cover of the restored coagulation capacity myelography may be performed. This was formerly done using oil contrast media but today water-soluble contrast media (Metrizamide; Amipaque, Nyegaard & Co AB, Oslo, Norway) should be used. Conventional myelography shows the level and extent of the compression. The radiologic appearance of the obstruction reveals whether the bleeding is extra- or intramedullary (Fig. 8.6). If there is total block of the passage of contrast medium, and if for surgical reasons it is necessary to assess the extent of the hematoma, lumbar as well as cervical puncture may be performed (Stanley and McComb 1983). In these cases water-soluble contrast media are preferable, as small amounts of contrast material may pass the block and provide enough concentration for a thorough CT examination (Pettersson and Harwood-Nash 1982). In the future, MRI may become of great value in these cases.

References

Abad Rico JM, Coello F, Alvarez F, Monasterio M (1979) Hematoma subarachnoideo espinal en la hemofilia B: descripcion de un caso y revision de la literatura. Rev Clin Esp 152: 479–483

Aledort LM (1976) The cause of death in hemophiliacs. In: Fratantoni JC, Aronson DL (eds) Unsolved therapeutic problems in hemophilia. US Department of Health, Education and Welfare (DHEW publication No (NIH) 77-1089), pp 9–14

Ambrose J (1973) Computerized transverse axial scanning (tomography), part 2. Clinical application. Br J Radiol 46: 1023–1047

Ambrose J (1974) Computerized axial scanning of the brain. J Neurosurg 40: 679–695

Bacher T (1980) Mortality among patients with haemophilia in Denmark during the period 1949–1978. Ugeskr Laeger 142: 1600–1603

Bruce DA, Schut L, Bruno LA, Wood JH, Sutton LN (1978) Outcome following severe head injuries in children. J Neurosurg 48: 679–688

Cromwell LD, Kerber C, Ferry P (1977) Spinal cord compression and hematoma; an unusual complication in a hemophilic infant. AJR 128: 847–849

Cronqvist S, Köhler R (1963) Angiography in epidural hematoma. Acta Radiol (Diagn) 1: 42–50

Cronqvist S, Brismar J, Kjellin K, Söderström CE (1975) Computed assisted axial tomography in cerebral vascular lesions. Acta Radiol (Diagn) 16: 13–45

Curless RG, Corrigan JJ Jr (1976) Headache in classical hemophilia: The risk of diagnostic procedures. Child's Brain 2: 187–194

de Villasante JM, Taveras JM (1976) Computerized tomography (CT) in acute head trauma. AJR 126: 765–778

Dolinskas C, Bilaniuk L, Zimmerman RA, Kuhl DE (1977) Computed tomography of intracerebral hematomas. I. Transmission CT observation on hematoma resolution. AJR 129: 681–688

Eyster ME, Gill FM, Blatt PM, Hilgartner MW, Bailard JO, Kinney TR, the Hemophilia Study Group (1978) Central nervous system bleeding in hemophiliacs. Blood 5: 1179–1188

Federici A, Minetti D, Grande C, Gatti L, Mannucci PM (1982) Intracranial bleeding in hemophilia: a study of eleven cases. Haematologica 67: 747–753

Forster G (1981) Role of the neurologist on the hemophilia comprehensive care team. Proc 2nd Int Symp Hemophilia Treatm, Tokyo, pp 17–20

Gore RM, Weinberger PE, Anandappa E, Shkolnik A, White H (1981) Intracranial complications of pediatric hematologic disorders: Computed tomographic assessment. Invest Radiol 3: 175–180

Greitz T, Lindgren E (1971) In: Abrams HL (ed) Angiography. Little, Brown and Company, Boston, pp 221–226

Harvie A, Lowe GDO, Forbes CD, Prentice CRM, Turner J (1977) Intraspinal bleeding in haemophilia: successful treatment with factor VIII concentrate. J Neurol Neurosurg Psychiatry 40: 1220–1223

Keely ML, Taylor N, Chard RL Jr (1972) Spinal cord compression as a complication of haemophilia. In: Gairnder D, Robinson R (eds) Arch Dis Child 47: 826–828

Kerr CB (1964) Intracranial hemorrhage in hemophilia. J Neurol Neurosurg Psychiatry 27: 166–173

Kinney TR, Zimmerman RA, Butler RB, Gill FM (1977) Computed tomography in the management of intracranial bleeding in hemophilia. J Pediatr 91: 31–35

Larsson SA, Wiechel B (1983) Deaths in Swedish hemophiliacs, 1957–1980. Acta Med Scand 214: 199–206

Levander B, Stattin S, Svendsen D (1975) Computed tomography of traumatic intra and extracerebral lesions. Acta Radiol (Suppl) 364: 107–118

Mamoli B, Sonneck G, Lechner K (1976) Intrakranielle und spinale Blutungen bei Hämophilie. J Neurol 211: 143–154

Matsuda M, Handa J, Asato R, Handa H, Yasunaga K (1977) Surgical treatment of intracranial hematoma and hydrocephalus in an infant with hemophilia A. Arch Surg Neurol 7: 199–203

McCarthy JW, Coble LL (1973) Intracranial hemorrhage and subsequent communicating hydrocephalus in a neonate with classical hemophilia. Pediatrics 51: 122–124

Moody RA, Mullan S (1968) Factor VIII in hemophilia: Case report. J Neurosurg 29: 520–523

New P, Scott W, Schnur J, Davis K, Taveras JM (1974) Computerized axial tomography with the EMI scanner. Radiology 110: 109–123

Newland AC, Walter PH, Wylie IG, Colvin BT (1979) The diagnosis of intracranial haemorrhage in haemophilia by computerized axial tomography. Clin Lab Haematol 1: 139–145

Omar MM, Binet EF (1978) Peripheral contrast enhancement in chronic epidural hematomas. J Comput Assist Tomogr 2: 332–335

Pettersson H, Harwood-Nash DC (1982) CT and myelography of the spine and cord. Springer, Berlin Heidelberg New York

Pettersson H, McClure P, Fitz C (1984) Intracranial hemorrhage in hemophilic children. Acta Radiol (in print)

Raggio JF, Fleischer AS, Corley CC (1978) Posterior fossa subdural hematoma in a hemophiliac. Neurosurgery 3: 213–215

Schiller F, Neligan G, Budtz-Olsen O (1948) Surgery in haemophilia: a case of spinal subdural haematoma producing paraplegia. Lancet II: 842

Seeler RA, Imana RB (1973) Intracranial hemorrhage in patients with hemophilia. J Neurosurg 39: 181–185

Silverstein A (1960) Intracranial bleeding in hemophilia. Arch Neurol 3: 141–157

Simpson DA, Robson HN (1960) Intracranial hemorrhage in disorders of blood coagulation. Aust NZ J Surg 29: 287–303

Stanley P, McComb JG (1983) Chronic spinal epidural hematoma in hemophilia A in a child. Pediatr Radiol 13: 241–243

Sumner DW (1962) Spontaneous spinal extradural hemorrhage due to hemophilia. Report of a case. Neurology 12: 501–502

Tellegen RJ (1850) Drie gevallen van bloederiziekte, waargenomen in Drenthe en Groningen. Nieuw praktisch Tijdschrift voor de Geneeskunde 2 (nieuwe reeks): 414–420

van Trotzenburg L (1975) Neurological complications of hemophilia. In: Brinkhous KM, Hemker HC (eds) Handbook of hemophilia. Excerpta Medica, Amsterdam, pp 389–404

Visconti EB, Hilgartner MW (1980) Recognition and management of central nervous system hemorrhage in hemophilia. Paediatrician 9: 127–137

Volpe JJ, Manica JP, Land VJ, Coxe WS (1976) Neonatal subdural hematoma associated with severe hemophilia A. Pediatrics 88: 1023–1025

Yoshida M, Hayashi T, Kuramoto S, Hiyoshi Y, Yokoyama T (1979) Traumatic intracranial hematomas in hemophiliac children. Surg Neurol 12: 115–118
Zouaoui A, Hirsch JF, Gazengel C, Pierre-Kahn A, Reiner D (1980) Les accidents neurologiques de l'hemophilie chez l'enfant. Neurochirurgie 26: 285–289

Chapter 9

The Neck and Chest

Bleeding into the sublingual, retropharyngeal, and paratracheal areas is a rare but potentially lethal complication that has been reported in both children and adults (Kitchens 1977; Pochedly and Rosales 1968). Early recognition is mandatory and may be life saving.

Severe intrathoracic hemorrhage has been described mainly in adults (Rasaretnam et al. 1976). This complication is uncommon, but several deaths have been described (Barrett and Israels 1965; Burke and Salzman 1959). In their examination of 118 deaths in hemophiliacs, Larsson and Wiechel (1983) found three patients who died from bleeding into the respiratory tract.

The Neck

Hemorrhage in the *retropharyngeal and paratracheal areas* is a dangerous complication (Biggs and McFarlane 1966; Edmond 1951). The extravasation of blood along the fascial planes surrounding the larynx, pharynx, and trachea may lead to increasing respiratory distress and asphyxia before the blood loss is significant (Pochedly and Rosales 1968). The early manifestation may be a "sore throat," and patients with such symptoms must be observed closely (Kitchens 1977). As the bleeding progresses, swelling and eventually ecchymoses may be apparent.

It is important to detect upper airway hemorrhage early in order to avoid complete obstruction and suffocation. The radiologic examination of the neck is valuable in this situation. In the lateral cervical radiograph, the normal retropharyngeal space (at C2) should not exceed 7 mm, and the retrotracheal space (at C6) 22 mm (Wholey et al. 1958). Retropharyngeal hematoma causes a widening of these spaces, with anterior displacement of the larynx, trachea, and esophagus (Kitchens 1977; Markowitz and Mendel 1981; McCook and Felman 1979). If the hematoma has dissected downwards into the thorax, the chest film may show a widening of the upper mediastinum. Use of CT has hitherto not been described in this condition, but today would be the method of choice for rapid and accurate evaluation.

The Chest

Hemomediastinum in hemophilia is very rare. It has been reported after minor trauma (Jivani and Mann 1970) and in association with bleeding in the neck from which blood tracked into the mediastinum (Edmond 1951; Pochedly and Rosales 1968). The combination of hemomediastinum and hemothorax has been described after emesis (Bart 1972).

The patients describe pain in the neck and shoulder, with stiffness of the neck. The pain is of gradual onset, worsened by deep breaths. If the bleeding is not controlled there might be swelling and bruising of the root of the neck after a few days, and the dyspnea may progress (Jivani and Mann 1970).

The radiologic plain film examination reveals a broadening of the mediastinum (Fig. 9.1), and possibly a deviation of the trachea. CT examination, which seems not to have been described in connection with hemomediastinum in hemophiliacs, reveals the nature of the broadening, as well as the exact extent of the mediastinal bleeding (Fig. 9.2). The CT examination is also of great value for control of the regression of the hematoma during treatment.

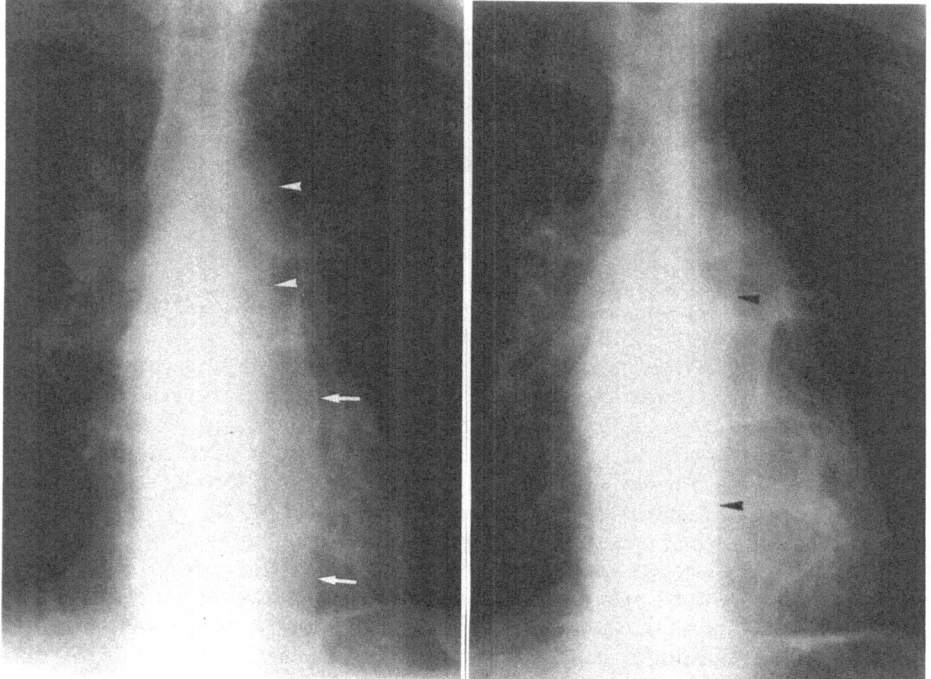

a   b

Fig. 9.1a,b. Hemomediastinum, conventional radiography. 23-year-old with severe hemophilia A. **a** Behind the heart, to the left of the descending aorta (*arrowheads*) there is an area of increased density with a sharp lateral demarcation (*arrows*). It is not possible to identify the thoracic aorta in its lower portion. The extension of the lesion to the right cannot be defined. **b** Same patient, conventional radiography 6 days later, following factor replacement therapy. The hematoma has resolved and is no longer visible. The descending aorta is visible in its whole thoracic extension (*arrowheads*).

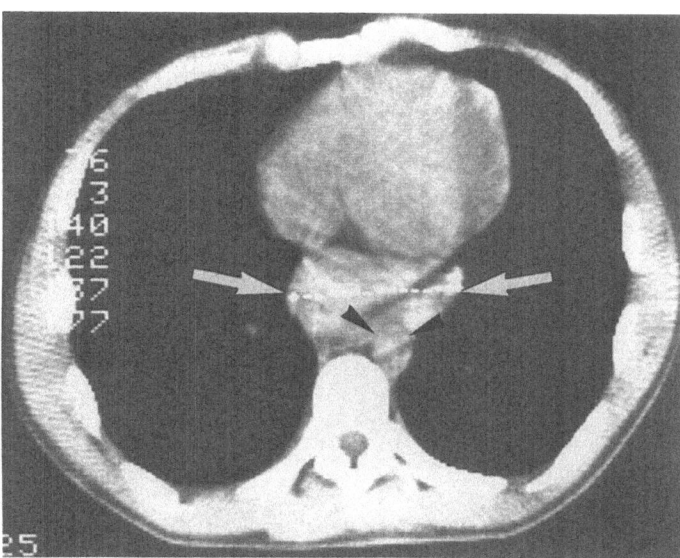

Fig. 9.2. Same patient and occasion as in Fig. 9.1a, CT. The mediastinal hematoma occupies the entire mediastinum between the heart and the vertebral column (*arrows*). There is clot formation in the hematoma, giving varying attenuation values. The anterior part of the aorta is embedded in the hemorrhage (*arrowhead*).

Spontaneous *hemothorax* has been reported only five times in the literature (Barrett and Israels 1965; Freedman et al. 1943; Kay and Kupfer 1957; Pendergrass and Neuhauser 1942; Rasaretnam et al. 1976). The hemothorax may also be caused by minor trauma (Barrett and Israels 1965; Jivani and Mann 1970) or may occur as a spontaneous *hemopneumothorax*, probably due to tearing of vascular adhesions at the rupture of superficial pleural blebs (Barrett and Israels 1965; Burke and Salzman 1959). The clinical symptoms consist of a sudden painful and tightening feeling in the chest, followed by more or less pronounced dyspnea. The pain is often worsened by coughing or sneezing (Barrett and Israels 1965).

The plain chest films reveal the hemorrhagic effusion (Fig. 9.3). Confirmation of the diagnosis may be made by needle aspiration under the cover of factor replacement. However, it can be done more safely by CT examination. The attenuation values of extravasated and clotted blood are higher than those of empyema or simple pleural effusion (Fig. 9.4).

Massive *intrapulmonary bleeding* is very rare and only scantily reported. One case described by Pursel and Sherman (1972) ended in pulmonary resection, while a massive pulmonary hemorrhage in a patient reported by Takeda and Mabuchi (1974) resulted in cavitation. The radiologic findings are not pathognomonic, and of course differential diagnoses such as pneumonia, tumor, and tuberculosis must be ruled out.

Minor pulmonary hemorrhage has been regarded as rare in the past, but in a review of the chest radiographs of 33 adult hemophiliacs Putman et al. (1976) found 12 patients with scarring, fibrosis, and pleural thickening consistent with sequelae of intrapulmonary bleeding or hemothorax. Such small bleedings may therefore be much more common than previously thought.

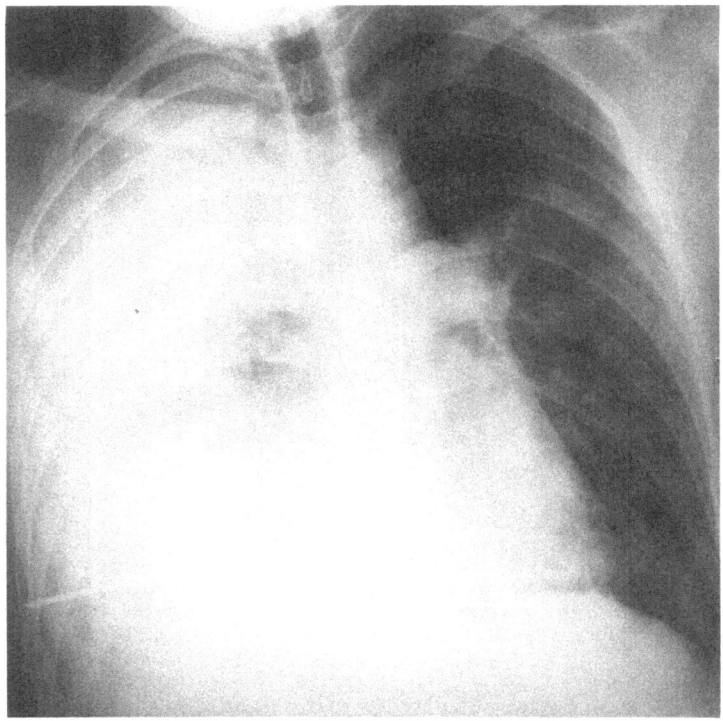

Fig. 9.3. Hemothorax, bedside examination. 22-year-old with severe hemophilia A. There is an extensive hemothorax occupying the main part of the right thoracic cavity.

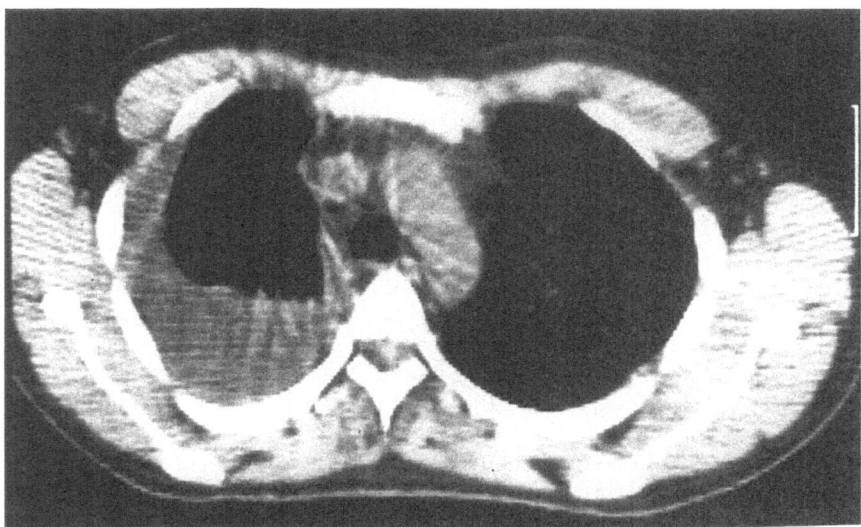

Fig. 9.4. Hemothorax, CT. 21-year-old with severe hemophilia A. The high attenuation value of the effusion confirms its hemorrhagic nature.

Spontaneous *hemopericardium* with cardiac tamponade has been described by Gaston et al. (1961) and Anderson (1964). Both patients had retrosternal pain, dyspnea, and signs of cardiac tamponade. Both were treated with factor replacement and recovered. The chest radiographs revealed massive enlargement of the heart shadow. CT can be used to differentiate this from a true cardiac enlargement or pericardial effusion.

Although muscle bleeding is common in hemophilia (Chap. 5), *myocardial bleeding* has not been reported, and in a survey of hemophilic boys aged 13–17 years, Thomas et al. (1976) could not find any signs of myocardial damage.

References

Anderson GA (1964) Spontaneous hemopericardium with cardiac tamponade and "pericardiotomy syndrome" complicating hemophilia. Am J Cardiol 13: 278–283

Barrett KE, Israels MCG (1965) Haemothorax in haemophilia. Thorax 20: 416–421

Bart JB (1972) Hemomediastinum and hemothorax in mild hemophilia. South Med J 65: 159–160

Biggs R, McFarlane RG (1966) Treatment of haemophilia and other coagulation disorders. Blackwell Scientific, Oxford

Burke JF, Salzman EW (1959) Spontaneous hemo-pneumothorax in a hemophiliac. JAMA 169: 1623–1625

Edmond AR (1951) Death from respiratory obstruction in hemophilia. Med J Aust 1: 227–228

Freedman P, Levine S, Solis-Cohen L (1943) Hemothorax in blood dyscrasias. Am J Med Sci 205: 692–696

Gaston LW, Mach BF, Beck WS (1961) Hemophilia A and concurrent factor VII deficiency. Studies of a patient with complicating cardiac tamponade. N Engl J Med 264: 1078

Jivani SKM, Mann J (1970) Haemomediastinum in a haemophiliac after minor trauma. Thorax 25: 372–374

Kay WR, Kupfer HG (1957) Spontaneous hemothorax in hemophilia; case report and discussion of the hemophilia syndromes with remarks on the management of hemothorax. Ann Int Med 47: 152–161

Kitchens CS (1977) Retropharyngeal hematoma in a hemophiliac. South Med J 70: 1421–1422

Larsson SA, Wiechel B (1983) Deaths in Swedish hemophiliacs, 1957–1980. Acta Med Scand 214: 199–206

Markowitz RI, Mendel JB (1981) Retropharyngeal bleeding in haemophilia. Br J Radiol 54: 521–523

McCook TA, Felman AH (1979) Retropharyngeal masses in infants and young children. Am J Dis Child 133: 41–43

Pendergrass EP, Neuhauser EBD (1942) Pleural lesions in haemophilia. AJR 48: 147–153

Pochedly C, Rosales A (1968) Respiratory obstruction in a child with classical hemophilia. Am J Dis Child 116: 103–105

Pursel SE, Sherman AK (1972) Pulmonary resection in hemophilia. Chest 62: 342–343

Putman CE, Gamsu G, Zuin D, McLoud T (1976) Radiographic chest abnormalities in adult hemophilia. Radiology 118: 41–43

Rasaretnam R, Chanmugam D, Sivathasan C (1976) Spontaneous haemothorax in a mild haemophiliac. Thorax 31: 601–603

Takeda R, Mabuchi H (1974) A massive pulmonary hemorrhage resulting in caviation occurring in a case of hemophilia A associated with diabetes mellitus. South Med J 67: 869–873

Thomas DJ, Fowler JM, Kirk P (1976) Letter: Myocardial bleeding in haemophilia. Br Med J II: 526

Wholey MH, Bruwer AJ, Baker HL Jr (1958) The lateral roentgenogram of the neck. Radiology 71: 350–356

Chapter 10

The Abdomen and Urinary Tract

Gastrointestinal hemorrhage occurs in about 20% of hemophiliacs (Dodds et al. 1970; Rose et al. 1981), mostly in older children and adults. Such bleeding may be serious and mortality is not uncommon (Dodds et al. 1970; Forbes et al. 1973). In Larsson and Wiechel's material (1983), 11 of 118 deaths in hemophiliacs were caused by bleeding into the gastrointestinal tract, and one by extensive hemorrhage into the greater omentum. Spontaneous splenic hemorrhage is very rare, only a few cases having been recorded, some with fatal outcome (Mariani et al. 1974; Stout et al. 1973; Thompson and Jackson 1974). Spontaneous liver bleeding has never been reported.

Bleeding into the urinary tract is common, being the most frequent clinical manifestation of hemophilia after hemarthrosis and soft tissue bleeding (Ramgren 1962; Rizza and Matthews 1972).

Gastrointestinal Tract

Clinical Aspects

As in any other patient group, gastrointestinal bleeding may be caused by gastric ulcers, ulcerative colitis, neoplasms, etc. The symptomatology and diagnostic imaging in these cases does not differ from that in other patients, and will not be discussed here. Apart from such bleeding, most of the hemophilic cases described in the literature had *intramural intestinal hemorrhage* with breakthrough into the intestinal lumen or more seldom into the peritoneal cavity (Khilnani et al. 1964; Lautkin et al. 1956; Rose et al. 1981). Bleeding is more common in the small intestine than in the colon (Harrison et al. 1972; Khilnani et al. 1964). It is rare in the stomach (Mahoney 1974) and has been described only once in the esophagus (Oldenburger and Gundlach 1977).

Diffuse hemorrhage in large areas of the wall of the bowel is the most common type of intramural hemorrhage in bleeding disorders (Eiland et al. 1978). Localized intramural hematomas in healthy individuals are usually produced by trauma but may be seen in hemophiliacs without preceding trauma (Eiland et al. 1978). Such localized hematomas may cause intestinal obstruction (Rose et al. 1981) or in rare instances act as the leading point of an intussusception (Fripp and Karabus 1977;

LeBlanc 1982). Depending on the site and the type of intramural bleeding, the patient may present with abdominal pain and distention, hematemesis, and melena or with the signs of intestinal obstruction.

Intramesenteric hemorrhage may be caused by overdistention of the stomach with tears of the small blood vessels in the lesser omentum. The blood may then track between the peritoneum and the posterior wall of the stomach, into the greater omentum (Adelman 1979). In the few cases of hemorrhage into the greater omentum described, the hematoma was localized, causing acute epigastrial pain with a palpable expansile lesion (Adelman 1979).

The acute abdomen in the hemophiliac may pose a difficult diagnostic problem in that it is necessary to differentiate hemorrhagic problems from other acute abdominal disorders. However, thorough interpretation of the clinical history and signs as well as of the radiologic findings permits accurate diagnosis in most cases (Dodds et al. 1970).

Diagnostic Imaging

In the diagnostic workup of *diffuse intramural hemorrhage* the preliminary plain films may reveal a paralytic ileus, and if the lumen of the affected area contains gas, narrowing of the lumen, scalloping, or thumb printing may be seen (Eiland et al. 1978). The appearance may be impossible to differentiate from ischemia of the bowel (Khilnani et al. 1964). The barium meal with gastrointestinal series usually reveals segmental affection, with narrowing of the lumen and thickening of

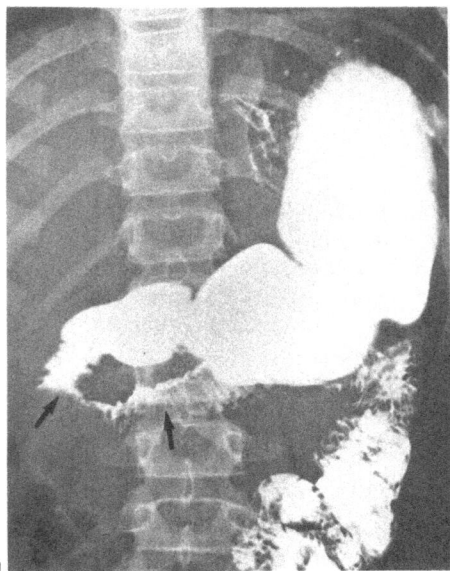 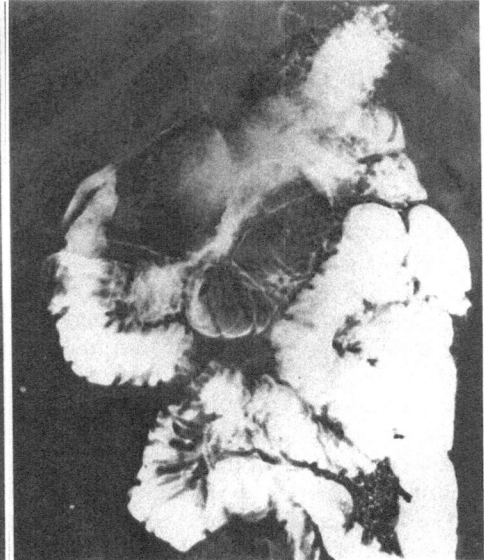

a   b

Fig. 10.1a,b. Diffuse intramural hemorrhage in the jejunum. Barium meal. **a** The lumen is heavily compressed over a long area, with thickening of the mucosal folds, which are sharply demarcated (*arrows*). **b** 3 weeks later, after conservative treatment, a repeat barium meal reveals a normal intestinal pattern.

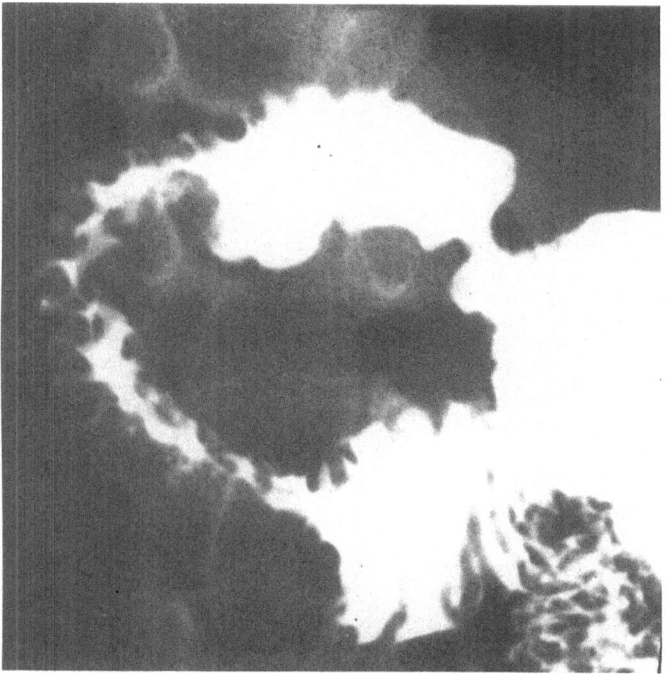

Fig. 10.2. Diffuse intramural hemorrhage of the duodenum. Barium meal. Slight trauma. The bowel is narrowed, and the wall is rigid with thumb printing.

the folds, which are sharply demarcated (Fig. 10.1). The bowel wall is rigid and thumb printing is common (Fig. 10.2). Barium enema of the colon reveals the same changes, but the folds and the thumb printing are larger than in the small bowel. Double contrast examination of the gastrointestinal tract provides detailed information but should not be performed in hemophiliacs with ongoing bleeding.

Large *localized intramural hematomas* bulge into the lumen and may cause total obstruction. The hematoma is sometimes visible on the plain films (Fig. 10.3a) and is well demonstrated on the upper gastrointestinal series (Fig. 10.4) or on barium enema of the colon (Fig. 10.3b) (Rose et al. 1981). The localized intramural masses are also well demonstrated on ultrasound examination and CT (Adelman 1979; Rose et al. 1981) (Fig. 10.5). If the hematoma causes intestinal obstruction, the barium meal may reveal only the dilated bowel and not the hematoma itself. During factor replacement therapy repeat barium meals or barium enemas may be used for evaluation of the resolution of the hemorrhage (Figs. 10.1b, 3c, 5c,d). In cases of localized hematomas, the healing can be followed by ultrasonography (Fig. 10.5d).

In suspected *intramesenteric hemorrhage*, with large localized hematomas, ultrasonography may give valuable information. However, the picture may be disturbed by bowel loops distended by gas. In such cases CT is the method of choice in that it not only shows the site and type of lesion but also its effect on neighboring structures (Fig. 10.6) (Adelman 1979). If a breakthrough into the intraperitoneal cavity is suspected, CT reveals the extent and localization of the blood collection.

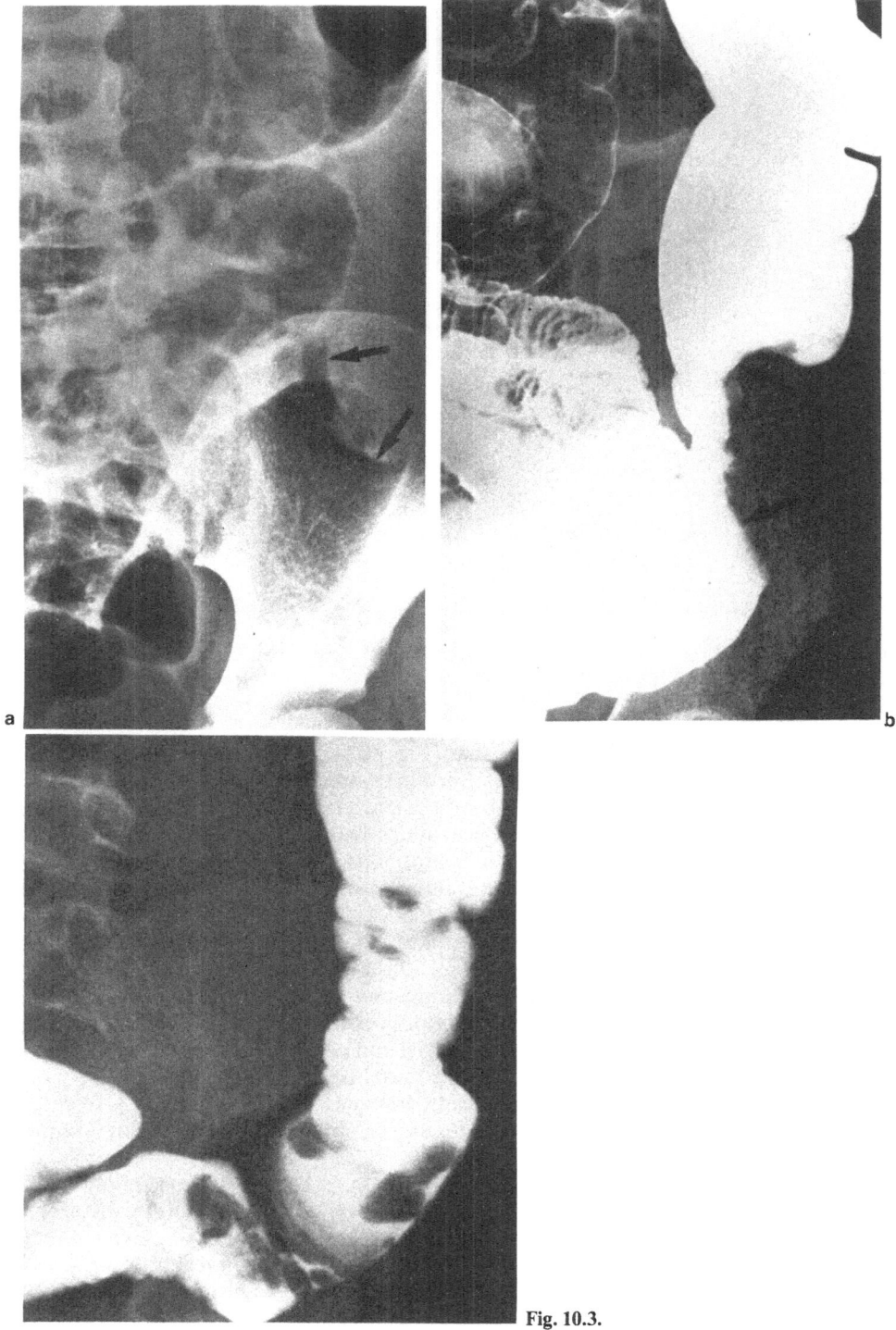

Fig. 10.3.

Fig. 10.3a–c. Localized intramural hematoma. 7-year-old with severe hemophilia A. No history of trauma. **a** On the plain film the hematoma may be seen bulging into the air-filled descending colon (*arrows*). **b** This finding is verified on the barium enema (*arrows*). **c** At repeat barium enema 3 weeks later, following factor replacement therapy, the hematoma has resolved. (By courtesy of F. Brunelle, MD, Hopital Bicetre, Paris, France)

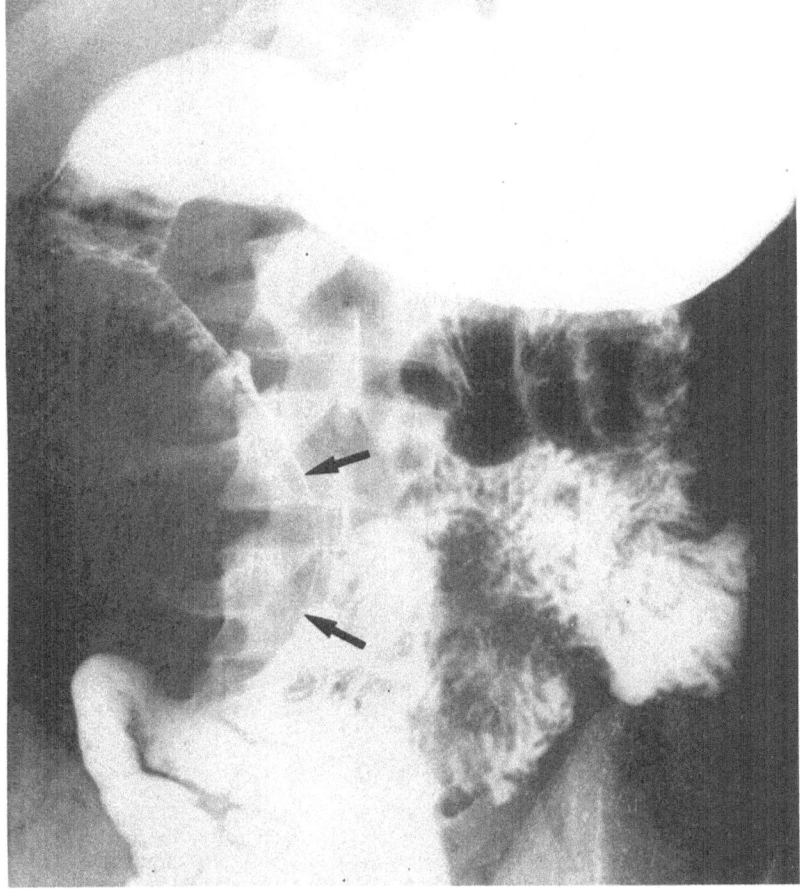

Fig. 10.4. Localized intramural hematoma, descending duodenum. 20-year-old with severe hemophilia A. No trauma. The large hematoma nearly totally obstructs the lumen. There is only a thin rim of barium (*arrows*) showing the passage to the bowel distal to the hematoma.

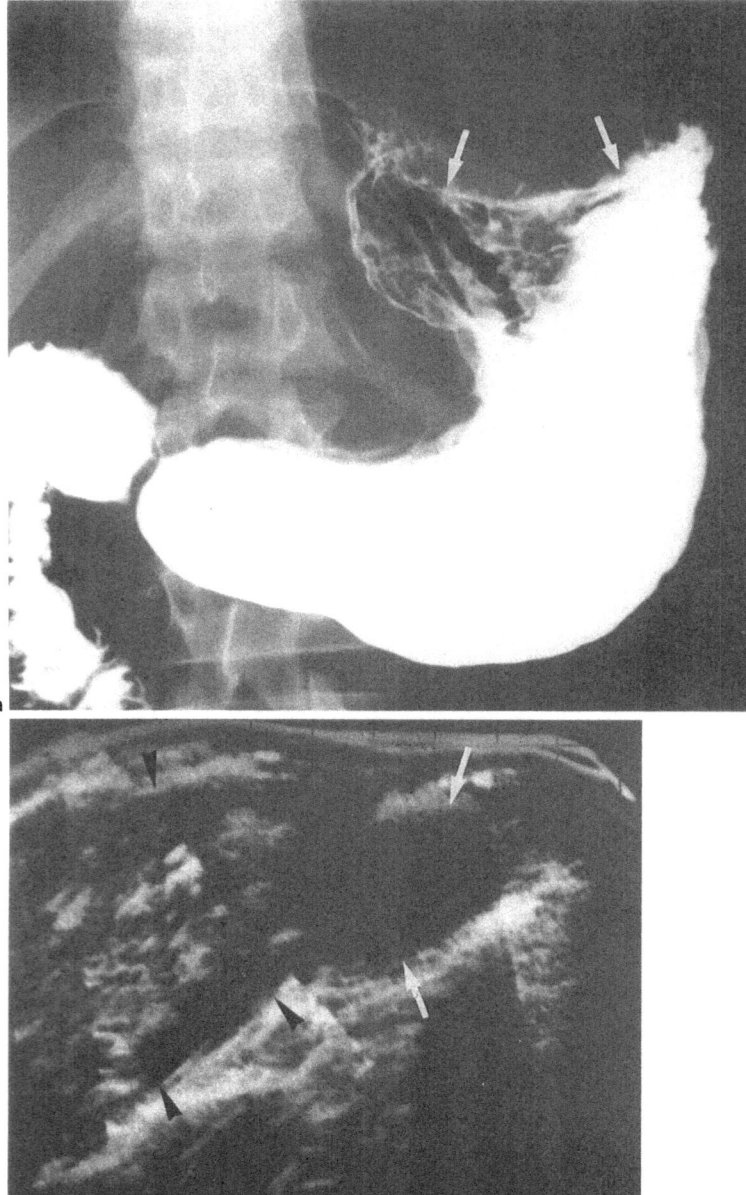

Fig. 10.5a–d. Localized intramural hemorrhage, conventional examination and ultrasonography. 22-year-old with severe hemophilia A. No trauma. **a,b** At the initial examination the barium meal (**a**) reveals a large expansile lesion compressing the fundus of the stomach (*arrows*). The border between the lesion and the stomach is irregular, with small streaks of barium contrast extending towards the lesion. This speaks in favor of an intramural hemorrhage as opposed to a hematoma outside the walls of the stomach. Ultrasonography at the same occasion (**b**) reveals the size and extent of the hematoma (*arrows*) and its close relation to the liver (*arrowheads*).

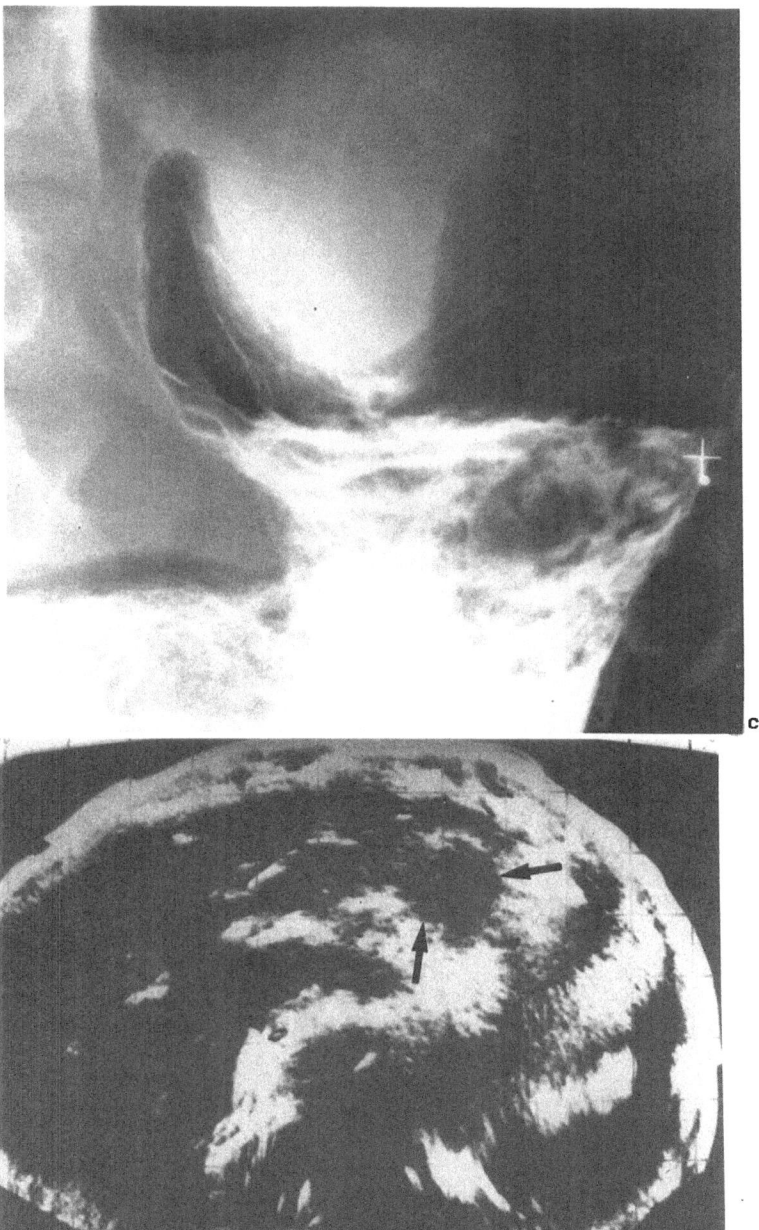

Fig. 10.5c,d. Repeat examination 4 weeks later during factor replacement therapy. The hematoma is considerably smaller, and its border towards the stomach is more smooth. The size and extent of the hematoma is clearly seen on both examinations (*arrows*).

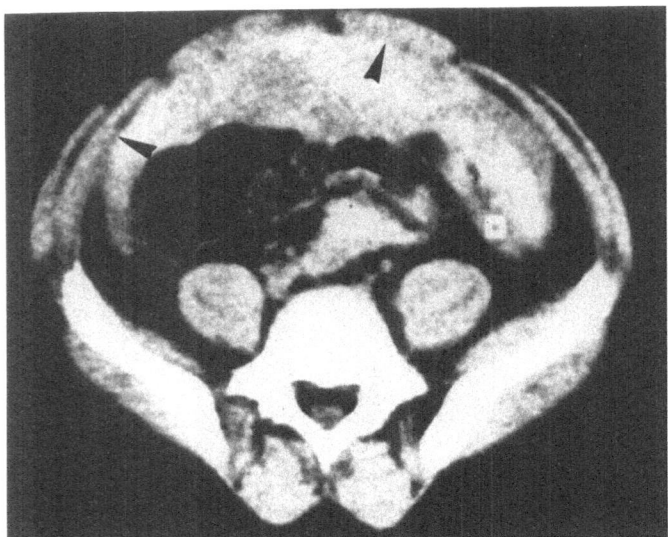

Fig. 10.6. Intramesenteric hemorrhage, CT. 14-year-old with severe hemophilia A. Minor trauma. There is a large hematoma in the mesentery, situated anteriorly in the abdomen. The hemorrhage does not involve the abdominal wall, as the CT reveals clear demarcation between the muscles of the wall and the hematoma (*arrowheads*). (By courtesy of A. Daneman, MD, the Hospital for Sick Children, Toronto, Canada)

Liver and Spleen

Splenic hematoma and rupture of the spleen are very rare in hemophiliacs but have been reported both after trauma (Gibson et al. 1976) and spontaneously (Mariani et al. 1974; Stout et al. 1973; Thompson and Jackson 1974). Some authors (Brook and Newman 1965; Gowda et al. 1968; Krauss and Hahn 1983) have postulated that their cases may have been caused by nausea and vomiting. Also one case of neonatal splenic hemorrhage, probably attributable to birth trauma, is on record (Iannaccone and Pasquino 1981).

In older children and adults, the symptoms have been right upper quadrant pain (Krauss and Hahn 1983), followed in some cases by shock if the bleeding is pronounced (Gibson et al. 1976).

The diagnostic imaging has previously included plain films of the abdomen, angiography (Stout et al. 1973), and scintimetry (Mariani et al. 1974), but today ultrasonography and CT are the methods of choice, giving detailed information on the status of the spleen as well as on possible intraperitoneal or retroperitoneal hemorrhage (Fig. 10.7).

Splenic rupture demands surgical intervention, and in the immediate postoperative period CT may be used to assess suspected recurrence of bleeding.

Ring-like calcifications have been reported as sequelae of intrasplenic hemorrhage (Innaccone and Pasquino 1981), and we have seen one case of scattered calcifications throughout the spleen (Fig. 10.8).

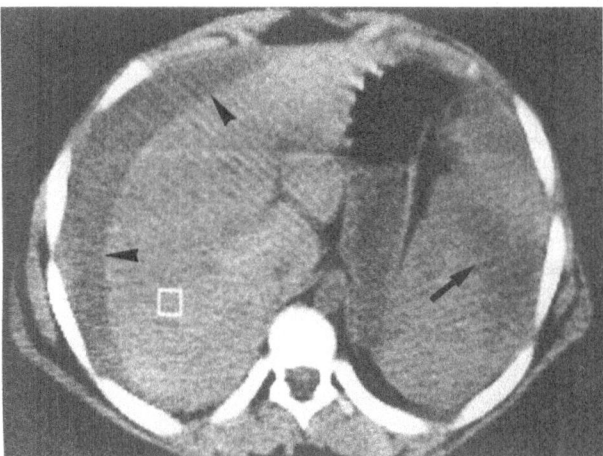

Fig. 10.7. Splenic hematoma and subcapsular liver hemorrhage, CT. 44-year-old with severe hemophilia A. Minor trauma. The spleen is enlarged and there are areas of decreased attenuation caused by hemorrhage (*arrows*). There is no breakthrough to the abdominal cavity, and the bleeding is kept within the splenic capsule. There is a large subcapsular liver hematoma (*arrowheads*) displacing the liver to the left. (By courtesy of A. Daneman, MD, the Hospital for Sick Children, Toronto, Canada)

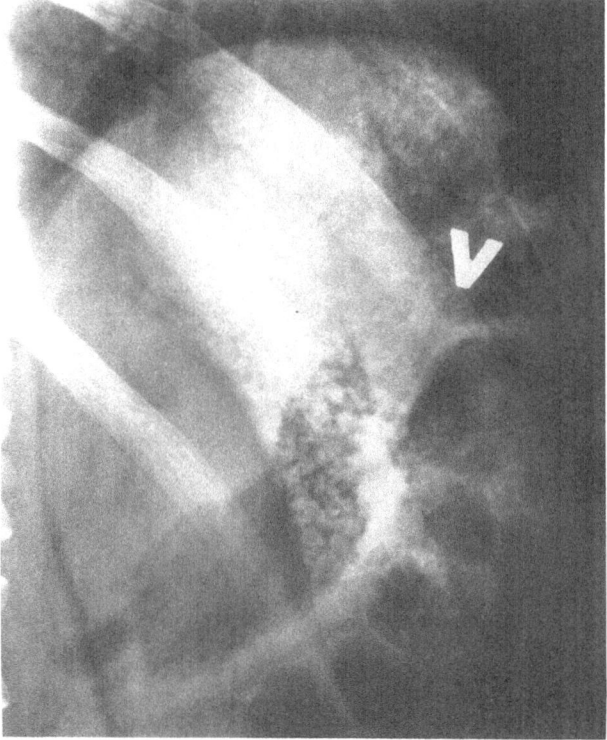

Fig. 10.8. Splenic calcifications. 28-year-old with severe hemophilia A. Numerous small calcifications throughout the spleen are the sequelae of intrasplenic hemorrhage.

Traumatic *rupture of the liver* in a hemophiliac is on record (English et al. 1976), but no spontaneous hemorrhage has hitherto been reported. *Hemobilia* after liver biopsy was reported by Elte et al. (1980) but spontaneous hemobilia has never been described. Again, ultrasonography and/or CT are the diagnostic modalities of choice. Although CT gives more detailed information (Fig. 10.7) ultra-sonography in most cases is quite sufficient and should be used for follow-up examinations during treatment (Fig. 10.9).

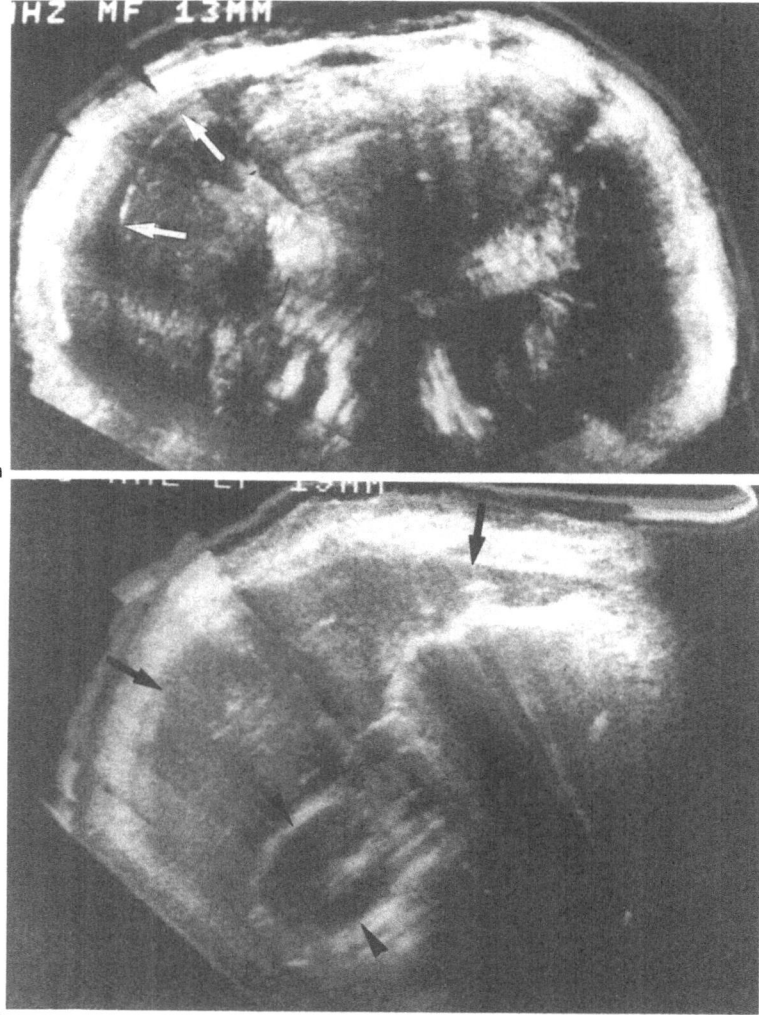

Fig. 10.9. Subcapsular liver hematoma, ultrasonographic examination. The same patient as in Fig. 10.7.
a Immediately after a minor trauma, there is an area of altered echogenicity between the abdominal wall and the liver. The border between the hematoma and the liver can be defined (*arrows*), cf. Fig. 10.7.
b 3 weeks later, after factor replacement therapy, the hematoma has resolved. There is no interposition of blood between the abdominal wall and the liver. The liver has normal echogenecity and is easy to define (*arrows*), as is the kidney (*arrowheads*).

The Urinary Tract

Bleeding into the urinary tract is rare in early childhood, but then increases rapidly in frequency and is common in adolescents (Davidson et al. 1949) as well as in adults. The bleeding is in most cases transient, disappearing without treatment. However, the hemorrhage may be persistent, causing anemia (Prentice et al. 1971). Deaths caused by bleeding per se are rare but some were reported before the era of modern replacement therapy (Forbes and Prentice 1977). Uremia, caused by calculi after repeated renal bleedings, is a known cause of death in hemophiliacs (Larsson and Wiechel 1983).

Clinical Aspects

A serious complication of hematuria is clot formation causing urinary obstruction (Blombäck and Nilsson 1958; Hilgartner 1966; Prentice et al. 1971). This clotting may seem paradoxical, but may be caused either by urinary thromboplastic activity or by effective factor replacement therapy. There are also reports of clot formation and renal obstruction after treatment with ε-aminocaproic acid (Hilgartner 1966; Stark et al. 1965).

Longstanding clots may calcify and patients with calcified stones have been recorded in most reports of renal abnormalities in hemophilia (Beck and Evans 1972; Dholakia and Howarth 1979; Prentice et al. 1971; Roberts et al. 1983; Waterfall 1981; Wright et al. 1971).

Obstructive uropathy and hydronephrosis may be caused not only by ureteric calculi but also by periureteric fibrosis. It has been suggested that such fibrosis may be caused by retroperitoneal hemorrhage (Beck and Evans 1972; Dholakia and Howarth 1979).

Renal papillary necrosis is a known complication of the hemoglobinopathies and has also been reported in the hemophilias (Beck and Evans 1972; Roberts et al. 1983). This papillary necrosis seems to run a benign course, apparently not affecting renal function (Roberts et al. 1983).

Intrarenal hematomas are rare, but both traumatic (Klamut et al. 1979) and spontaneous bleedings are on record (Dholakia and Howarth 1979). Intramural bleeding in the ureter has been reported in a single case (Patriquin 1980), as has traumatic rupture of the ureter (Forbes et al. 1971).

Diagnostic Imaging

In the diagnostic workup of the lesions of the urinary tract intravenous urography is suitable in most situations. This examination must be performed without any external compression of the ureters. The urogram reveals any obstruction present and possibly its cause, e.g., calculi or periureteral fibrosis (Fig. 10.10). In addition the degree of hydronephrosis and the influence on the renal pelvis and the ureter of intrarenal or retroperitoneal masses are delineated (Dholakia and Howarth 1979). The damage to the renal calyces is easily assessed in cases of renal papillary necrosis (Roberts et al. 1983).

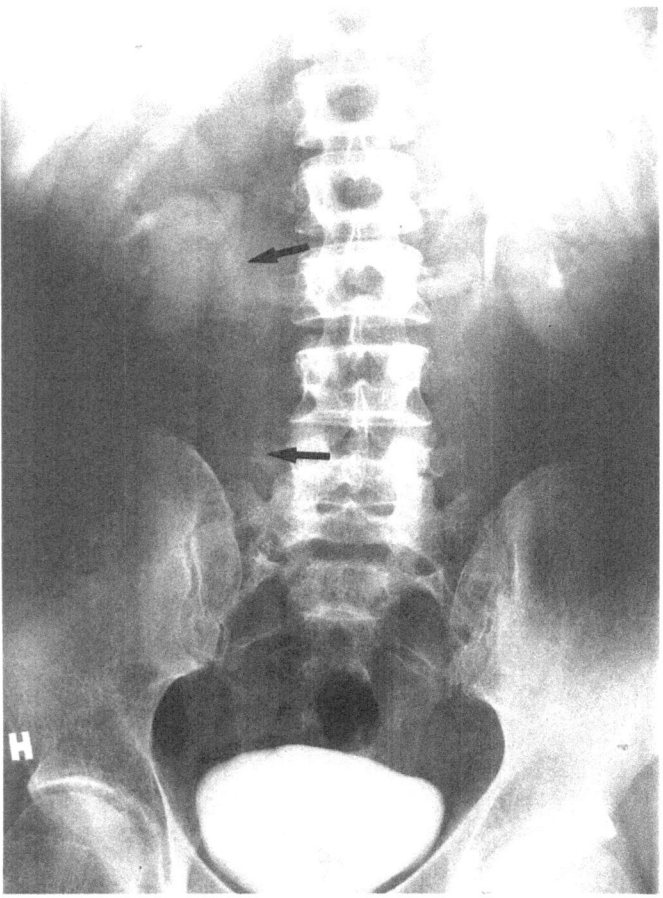

Fig. 10.10. Urinary obstruction, intravenous urography. 35-year-old with severe hemophilia A. A blood clot is situated in the right ureter, causing obstruction (as later verified at cystoscopy). The clot is not visible on the urogram, but the ureter and the renal pelvis are moderately dilated proximal to the obstruction (*arrows*).

However, if hydronephrosis or intrarenal masses are suspected, or if the renal function is impaired, ultrasonographic examination should be the diagnostic method of choice. For detailed assessment of intrarenal and periureteral masses CT is superior.

It should be stressed that although hematuria in hemophiliacs is a common symptom and often neglected by the patient, it must not be overlooked by the physician. Intravenous urography should be performed following the first episode and after frequent recurrence (Barkagan et al. 1974; Klement et al. 1978). Reasons for hematuria other than hemophilia may be found, and obstruction with slowly developing deterioration of renal function may occur even in patients who have noticed only a few episodes of hematuria (Prentice et al. 1971).

References

Adelman MI (1979) Localized intramesenteric haemorrhage—a recognisable syndrome in haemophilia? Br Med J 15: 642–643

Barkagan ZS, Linkina AI, Bishevsky KM (1974) Hematuric syndrome in hemophilia—characteristics of its development, clinical course and therapy. Ter Arkh 8: 99–106

Beck P, Evans KT (1972) Renal abnormalities in patients with haemophilia and Christmas disease. Clin Radiol 23: 349–354

Blombäck M, Nilsson IM (1958) Treatment of hemophilia A with human antihemophilic globulin. Acta Med Scand 161: 301–308

Brook J, Newman PE (1965) Spontaneous rupture of a spleen in hemophilia. Arch Intern Med 115: 595–597

Davidson CS, Epstein RD, Miller GF, Tailer FHL (1949) Hemophilia. A clinical study of 40 patients. Blood 4: 97–119

Dholakia AM, Howarth FH (1979) The urinary tract in haemophilia. Clin Radiol 30: 533–538

Dodds WJ, Spitzer RM, Friedland GW (1970) Gastrointestinal roentgenographic manifestation of hemophilia. AJR 110: 413–416

Eiland M, Han SY, Hicks GM Jr (1978) Intramural hemorrhage of the small intestine. JAMA 239: 139–142

Elte PM, van Aken WG, Agenant DMA, Tijtgat GN (1980) Hemobilia after liver biopsy. Early detection in a patient with mild hemophilia A. Arch Intern Med 160: 839–840

English PJ, Sheppard EM, Wensley RT (1976) Traumatic rupture of the liver in a haemophilic patient with factor VIII inhibitors. Lancet I: 1299–1300

Forbes CD, Prentice CRM (1977) Renal disorders in hemophilia A and B. Scand J Hematol 30: 43–50

Forbes CD, Craig JA, Prentice CRM, McNicol GP, Levack JH, Ireland JT, Adams JF, Sutherland GR (1971) Rupture of the ureter due to crushing injury in a boy with severe haemophilia. Br J Surg 58: 931–934

Forbes CD, Barr RD, Prentice RM, Douglas AS (1973) Gastrointestinal bleeding in haemophilia. Q J Med 42: 503–511

Fripp RR, Karabus CD (1977) Intussusception in haemophilia: a case report. S Afr Med J 52: 617–618

Gibson B, Wright FW, Rizza CR, Dudley NE (1976) Late successful treatment of splenic rupture in a haemophilic boy. Br Med J I: 260–262

Gowda M, Vietti T, Ternberg JL (1968) The use of cryoprecipitate in the surgical treatment of spontaneous rupture of the spleen in a hemophilia patient. Surgery 64: 1019–1020

Harrison HC, Lord RSA, Chesterman CN, Biggs JC, Tracy GD (1972) Spontaneous intramural haematoma in the sigmoid colon of a haemophiliac. Aust NZ J Surg 42: 69–70

Hilgartner M (1966) Intrarenal obstruction in haemophilia. Lancet I: 486

Iannaccone G, Pasquino AM (1981) Calcifying splenic hematoma in a hemophilic newborn. Pediatr Radiol 10: 183–185

Khilnani MT, Marshak RH, Eliasoph J, Wolff BS (1964) Intramural intestinal hemorrhage. AJR 92: 1061–1071

Klamut M, Szcerbo-Trojanowska M, Kowalewski J, Nowakowski A (1979) Transcatheter embolization in a haemophiliac with post-traumatic renal haemorrhage. Report of a case. Acta Radiol 20: 606–608

Klement AA, Fedorova ZD, Volkova SD, Papayan LP, Kuzmin DS, Klimenchenko GA, Egorova LV, Lapin AA (1978) Clinico-roentgenological characteristics of renal hemorrhage in hemophilia. Vestn Khir 121: 99–103

Krauss IS, Hahn DA (1983) Hemophilic splenic rupture without thrombocytosis. South Med J 24: 272–274

Larsson SA, Wiechel B (1983) Deaths in Swedish hemophiliacs. Acta Med Scand 214: 199–206

Lautkin A, Korelitz BI, Berger L (1956) Roentgen findings in the colon in a hemophiliac with melena. J Mt Sinai Hosp 23: 319–323

LeBlanc KE (1982) Jejuno-jejunal intussusception in a hemophiliac: A case report. Ann Emerg Med 11: 149–151

Mahoney DH (1974) Intramural gastric lesion with sudden abdominal pain. JAMA 230: 603–604

Mariani G, Ziparo V, De Rossi G, Boehmig P, Crisculolo D, Lombardi M, Scopinaro F (1974) Spontaneous splenic haematoma in haemophilia. Report of a case and review of the literature. Haematologica (Pavia) 59: 205–211

Oldenburger D, Gundlach WJ (1977) Intramural esophageal hematoma in a hemophiliac. An unusual cause of gastrointestinal bleeding. JAMA 237: 800

Patriquin H (1980) Ureteric hemorrhage in hemophilia with rapid healing. J Can Assoc Radiol 31: 265–266

Prentice CMR, Lindsay RM, Barr RD, Forbes CD, Kennedy AC, McNicol GP, Douglas AS (1971) Renal complications in haemophilia and Christmas disease. Q J Med, New Series XL, 157: 47–61

Ramgren O (1962) Hemophilia in Sweden. Acta Med Scand 171: 237

Rizza CR, Matthews JM (1972) Management of the hemophilic child. Arch Dis Child 47: 451–455

Roberts GM, Evans KT, Bloom AL, Al-Gailini F (1983) Renal papillary necrosis in haemophilia and Christmas disease. Clin Radiol 34: 201–206

Rose J, Hertz I, Weinberg B, Leleiko N, Harris MD (1981) Duodenal radiographic findings in hemophilia. Am J Gastroenterol 76: 160–165

Stark SN, White JG, Langer L Jr, Krinit W (1965) Epsilon-amino-caproic acid therapy as a cause of intrarenal obstruction in hematuria of hemophiliacs. Scand J Haematol 2: 97–107

Stout C, Hampton JW, Anderson JD, Oruc N (1973) Fatal nontraumatic splenic rupture in hemophilia and the Kasabach Merritt Syndrome. South Med J 66: 791–795

Thompson DS, Jackson JM (1974) Letter: Splenectomy in haemophilia. Med J Aust 1: 413

Waterfall WB (1981) Bilateral renal stones in a haemophiliac. Br J Urol 53: 481

Wright FW, Matthews JM, Brock LG (1971) Complications in hemophilic disorders affecting the renal tract. Radiology 98: 571–576

Subject Index

CT and Myelography of the Spine and Cord

Techniques, Anatomy and Pathology in Children

By **H. Pettersson, D. C. F. Harwood-Nash**
In association with C. R. Fitz and S. Chuang

1982. 93 figures. XIII, 119 pages. ISBN 3-540-11322-3

"This small textbook ... very effectively defines the role of computerized tomographic (CT) metrizamide-enhanced myelography in the evaluation of the pediatric patient. ... (The authors) found that CT-metrizamide myelography offered additional information in a sufficiently large number of instances to recommend it routinely as a supplement to conventional metrizamide myelograms. The book is a worthy addition to the shelves of institutions where children with spinal diseases are studied."
Dennis Osborne
Journal of Neurosurgery

"I belive the authors have achieved their goal of presenting a complete and concise presentation of the technique of CT metrizamide myelography. The book will benefit all physicians in the neurosciences who deal with pediatric diseases of the spine and spinal cord and can be recommended for this group."
Frederick S. Vines
American Journal of Roentgenology

"Though this textbook is small, it is absolutely full of information and gives an excellent account of combined water soluble contrast myelography and CT scanning in children. The illustrations are of excellent quality and there is quite extensive bibliography. The text contains valuable information for both technical and diagnostic personnel and is recommended without reservation for those monitoring CT; and departments who are not in the privileged position of having CT available, but who are monitoring a myelographic service."
G. T. Vaughan
Paraplegia

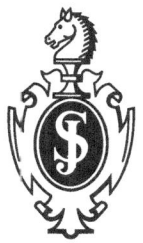

Springer-Verlag
Berlin
Heidelberg
New York
Tokyo

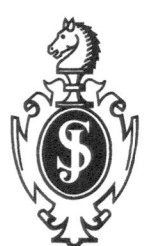